woman to woman

a guide to lesbian sexuality

Carol Booth

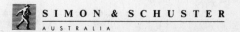
SIMON & SCHUSTER
AUSTRALIA

First published in Australia in 2002 by
Simon & Schuster (Australia) Pty Limited
20 Barcoo Street, East Roseville NSW 2069

A Viacom Company
Sydney New York London

National Library of Australia
Cataloguing-in-Publication data

Booth, Carol
    Woman to woman: a guide to lesbian sexuality.

    Bibiography.
    Includes index.
    ISBN 0 7318 0953 X.

    1. Sex instructions for lesbians. 2. Lesbians - Sexual behaviour.
    I. Title.

306.7663

Cover design: Gayna Murphy GREENDOT
Cover photograph: Austral Images
Author photograph courtesy of *Australian Doctor*, photographer Stefan Moore
Internal design: Avril Makula GRAVITY AAD
Typeset in Berkeley Book 10.5 pt on 14 pt
Printed in Australia by Griffin Press

10 9 8 7 6 5 4 3 2 1

Contents

Acknowledgments

For their professional help and advice: Dr Helen O'Connell (for reading and editing Chapter 2), Sarah Bergin and Dr Alison Rutherford (for reading and editing Chapter 5), Jen Rudland, Liz Hammond (for reading and editing Chapter 12, and her comments that helped shape Chapter 13 and several other chapters). Chetane, Gail and Libby of the Feminist Bookshop, Carina, Tim, Sinead and Anne, Michelle (from 2010), Cristina Garduño Freeman, who answered my cry for help and produced diagrams at an hour's notice, and Edwina Riddell, who took my hand-drawn efforts and made them into intelligible drawings.

For the many women who contributed their stories and comments, including: Margaret, Silva, Bev, Miah, Michelle, Narelle, Jac, Sarah, Jan, Melissa, Delece, Tania, Annie, Kerrie, Sue, Jude, Karen, Lisa, Geraldine, Claire, Louise, Sam and Fiona, Judith, Julie, Zoe, Hannah, Helen, Tracey, Jean, Jules, Sandra and Melanie.

For my friends, who read countless drafts, made suggestions and cups of tea, and who generously and unrestrainedly told me their stories. Some answered telephone calls that began '...Help, I'm stuck, tell me about your orgasms...", and others loved me and still kept inviting me to dinners and gatherings even though I'd been saying 'I can't come, I have to write' for years! Deb, Sylvia, Bev, Wendy, Liz, Nerida, Cath, Cassandra, Sarah, Katja, Alison, Kim, Fiona, Leanne, Lotus, Jan. And to those who have always been there for me: Keith Seckold, Jo Byrnes and Sam Goodwin.

To Brian, Ailsa and Jane, whose practical support made life possible.

To Alison and Dale for candlelight, photography and much astute comment.

To those women whom I may have known only in passing, but who have been role models and who have in one way or another shaped the lesbian woman I have become: Virginia, Heather and Helen, Lavender, Sand, Jan, Kerryn and Denise.

And to Julie Stanton, Clare Wallis and Jody Lee at Simon & Schuster for their expertise in bringing it all together.

Dedication

To my mum Terry, and my sister Brenda, for your unending support. For rescuing me when I had pneumonia, for cups of tea when I was heartbroken, for financial support, for your continuing belief that this book would actually be published. Brenda, for dropping everything and making scores of phone calls to check the accuracy of the resources section. For all the 'white light' and for the limitless love you both have showered on me. Dedicated with deepest thanks, and all the love my heart can hold.

To Leah, who encouraged me to gain the computer skills that allowed me to begin, and who supported my early efforts. Just as from the first, you were confident this would be published, I hold the vision of you fulfilling your potential for leadership and creativity. I see you embracing all that you can be. Dedicated with warmth and goodwill. For the good times!

Introduction
(or, is this book really necessary?)

This book was born one night at the dinner table. We had four women guests. Two friends were 'straight'[1] doctors. The other two guests were a lesbian couple. One of the heterosexual doctors became engrossed in an American book titled *Lesbian Sex* and faded from the conversation.

When the others commented on her lack of interest in our discussion, she said, 'A women came to see me recently. She said she thought she must be lesbian or at least bisexual. She had met someone and felt they might soon be in a relationship. She came to see me for sex education. She asked about safe sex and what lesbians did in bed.'

'What did you tell her?' I asked.

'I didn't have a clue what to say.'

Another straight friend said, 'Lesbian sex is just sort of mutual masturbation isn't it?'

Well, it is and it isn't. That description prompts most lesbian women to expressions of outrage. It leaves out the essence of lesbian sex, the colour and vibrancy of women making love with each other.

That night I decided that this book had to be written! Australian women needed a resource!

It seems strange to me now that any two people who wanted to have sex with each other would not know what to do. However, I remember that about fourteen years ago, I was puzzling over exactly the same issue. When I turned thirty, the long relationship with my man was ending. I was wondering what sort of relationship I would have next. I had close friendships with a number of lesbian women. I spent long hours staring out of the window of my commuter train, fantasising about women I was attracted to. I would imagine how women might behave in bed, and think, 'I'm sure that's what they must do.' Then I would be beset by doubt: 'Have I really got it right?'

My doubt was compounded by my friends' jokes: 'All we really do is hold hands', and 'Lesbians don't do anything. That's why Queen Victoria didn't make us illegal.' Like most heterosexual couples, my acquaintances did not discuss the details of their bedroom practices. When I went hunting, the local library yielded only a few dusty books on lesbian feminism. Finding accurate sexual information was not easy.

So when I heard our friend's dinner table story, this book was born. Knowledge about lesbian sex is not just for women who identify as lesbian. This is a century of new values and self-exploration. All women need to know the full range of their options.

It's true that if the woman who went to see our friend for sex education had instead gone home to bed, cuddled up with her partner, and investigated, she would have discovered the basics of lesbian sex. But why should it be so difficult? Let's face it, there have been 'how to' manuals about heterosexual sex around for years.

This book, therefore, is not only for Australian lesbians but also for all women who are interested in exploring the lesbian part of their sexuality. I am a lesbian and a doctor, but I do not feel that I am an expert on lesbian sex. The lesbian universe is a rich and diverse one. I accept at the outset that anything I present can only come with my particular flavour. That flavour is unashamedly, vivaciously, variously vanilla! I've learned a lot from the women who have contributed to this book, and I'm sure I've got heaps more to learn! At all times, except where I've directly quoted someone, this book is just my view. If you are a lesbian woman reading these pages, and you feel, 'That's not what it's like for me!', I would invite you to write to me. Let me know the way in which I incorrectly represented your world.

I have tried to write simply and, as far as possible, not to use technical terms. I have tried to stay away from political comment. I have also tried to be as direct and sexually explicit as I know how to be. I am aware of the possibility of offending some women by blunt language. However, it is not my intention to shock or offend; rather, it is my intention to make the ideas and practices of lesbian sexuality and relationship accessible.

In the book many women have told their stories. These are in italics. Many of these accounts are taken directly from conversations or interviews with individual women who have given permission for their words to be used. If the woman has given permission for me to do so, I have used her true first name. If she has preferred to remain anonymous I have used a different name to protect her privacy. Many experiences are common to a large number of women. I have been told very similar stories over and over again by different women. For this reason, some of the quotes are composites.

Below I have told my story. because who I am influences how I see the world.

I first remember being attracted to women whilst I was in relationship with a long-term male partner. We would be walking down the street and he would notice women he was attracted to. He'd say something to me like, 'Hasn't she got a gorgeous backside?' In those days, I didn't want him to see that this upset me. So I'd say, 'Yeah, great boobs too!' One day, I remember thinking, 'My God, she has got a great backside'. I credit my guy for drawing my attention to the sensual and sexual qualities of women.

Some time later, I remember hearing about lesbians. Before then, the concept of women loving women had never crossed my mind. After I heard about the idea, I mentioned it to my mother. She said, 'Well, it makes sense that a woman would know, better than a man, what a woman wants and needs'. Goddess bless my mum. I later learned that this concept is called 'gender empathy'.

Time passed, and I found myself on a management committee with a number of lesbian women. At first, I was scared of them. They seemed so unlike me. They were strong and confident, and didn't appear to care what people thought. They didn't wear the same clothes or make-up. I felt as if we were from different worlds.

Over time we all became friends. I joined reading and music groups with them. For a long time, I never thought about what they did in bed, they were just my friends. Then my relationship began to flounder and I started thinking about the future. It dawned on me that whilst I was obviously capable of heterosexuality, I was also attracted to women. Talk about being thrown into a spin, it felt like my world was fragmenting. You need to realise that I didn't know any public figures who were lesbian icons then.

I had heard about a book called Lesbian Sex by JoAnn Loulan. I phoned The Feminist Bookshop in Lilyfield, and quoted my bankcard number over the phone. I didn't want the book sent to my home. The woman at the shop suggested that they wrap it in two layers of brown paper and post it to my workplace. The book arrived at my very proper legal office. I finished work early that day and drove my car up to a lookout high on the cliffs overlooking Newcastle. Within three hours I had read the book cover to cover. I felt as if I had come home.

If my book can do something similar for just one woman it will have achieved my purpose.

I would like to acknowledge my debt to JoAnn Loulan. Her book helped me to start my lesbian life. Later on, her book inspired me to write. JoAnn was writing for lesbians. (Her book is still available and The Feminist Bookshop is still in the telephone directory.) Now I believe that *all* women, as they investigate who they are, may be interested in the contents of these pages. I hope you enjoy this book and that it either gives affirmation to what you do and who you are, or opens up ideas and universes for you.

With love
Carol Booth
Email: carolbooth@gay.com
November 2001

1

Women's Sexuality

P atterns of sexual behaviour have changed radically in the last thirty years, with people in Western countries becoming both more sexual and more sensual.[1] The sexual revolution, which began in the 1960s, was part of a changing consciousness that questioned all existing social values. At around the same time a new feminist movement began. Although many of our grandmothers remained confined to their roles as wives and mothers, individual women started to explore the world outside their homes. For some, this included an exploration of their sexuality. A few women had the courage to express what they learned about sex and sensuality in art and literature. However, little of their art or literature ever became available to other women.[2]

Women have been exploring their sexuality with increasing freedom. Although public acknowledgment and awareness of lesbianism have changed over the centuries, about ten per cent of women have always been exploring their sexuality with each other.[3]

Lesbian women[4] have always pushed the boundaries. In being true to ourselves, we have stepped outside culturally acceptable limits of sexual and social behaviour. However, by our presence and courage in allowing ourselves to be seen, we have been part of the force of social change.

> **CHRIS:** *Watching how Virginia behaved at work was great for me. When people assumed her partner was a man, she would quietly let them know that wasn't the case. She was fantastic. At first some workers gave her a hard time behind her back. But she stayed. She was good at her job. People changed. They liked her and respected her. Knowing her gave me the freedom to acknowledge that I was a dyke too.*[5]

With the realisation that variety brings richness to life, Australian culture is now much more accepting of diversity. Increased migration to Australia from Europe and Asia after the Second World War allowed Australians the opportunity to try many new foods. They slowly learned about other cultures, and noticed that what they learned was interesting, useful and enjoyable. Homosexuality is another new frontier for our culture. Many women are curious about lesbian sex, lesbian lifestyle and lesbian culture.

The 1990s saw lesbian women becoming much more visible. And these days, almost every woman's magazine has a story about a lesbian or lesbian relationship. Many television programs now have gay or lesbian characters. It has become 'chic' to be lesbian.

Despite current mainstream acceptance, it is important to realise that lesbian sexuality is not new. The social acceptability of lesbianism has waxed and waned over time, but lesbian relationships have existed among all peoples and throughout all ages.[6]

A brief 'herstory'[7]

Perhaps the most well-known lesbian of early times was the lyrist Sappho, who lived on the Greek island of Lesbos in the sixth and fifth centuries BC. She lived in a colony of women, and her poems and songs honoured their love for each other. In her own lifetime, Sappho's poetry was known throughout the Greek world. 'No woman of her time was more celebrated.'[8] Coins were minted with her face on them.

It was not until hundreds of years later (around 380AD) that her work began to be derided. When the Roman Emperors accepted Christianity, the 'ridicule of Sappho turned to censure'.[9] At this time male homosexuality was made a criminal offence, punishable by death, and Sappho's poetry was collected and publicly burned.

During the Renaissance, some of her lyrics were recovered, and again she was held in high esteem. However, it is said that her work was burned a second time in eleventh century Europe.[10] Only fragments of her work remain available today.

Just as Sappho's poetry has spiralled through acceptability and public contempt, so has lesbianism. In the sixteenth century the term 'donna con donna' was used in France to describe lesbian lovemaking. It was considered to be a harmless frivolity,[11] but by 1700 attitudes had changed, with descriptions such as 'this filthy vice' being used.[12] In the eighteenth century 'romantic friendship' between women was not only condoned but encouraged.[13] These friendships were intense and passionate. Couples shared '...one bed, one board and one purse'.[14] Eleanor Butler and Sarah Ponsonby were Irish women who eloped with each other in 1778 to live in Llangollen. They lived together, and shared their bed, for fifty years.[15] The sexual nature of their friendship was speculated on in the newspapers of the day.[16] However, their relationship was considered '...not only socially permissible but even desirable'.[17] They were role models for lesbian women of their era, and from that time forward.[18] Such relationships between women were not at all uncommon. Their sensuality did not always involve genital sex, but the physical expression of passion, including kissing, caressing and fondling, was normal. Hugging and kissing between women in public was acceptable.[19]

Late in the nineteenth century, 'Boston Marriages' were well known in the United States. They were usually long-lasting, committed, monogamous relationships between two women. Women in these relationships were frequently feminists, always independent of men, and generally lived together. There was usually no public acknowledgment regarding whether or not the relationships involved genital sexuality. However, a contemporary male journalist of the era described Boston marriages as '…a union – there is no truer word for it'.[20] In the Paris of 1900, lesbianism was fashionable. Natalie Barney and Renée Vivien were the centre of a group of artists, writers and poets. Barney founded her famous 'salon', which was visited by the most eminent women artists of the time. It was said that Barney had 'established a kind of Lesbos in Paris'.[21] Visitors to the salon included the celebrated author Gertrude Stein and her partner of thirty-eight years, Alice B. Toklas, as well as the English author Vita Sackville West, who was Virginia Woolf's lover.

However, around the time of the First World War, views began to change. It has been suggested that this changing attitude to lesbianism was partly due to emerging medical theories about the cause of homosexuality, and also to the fact that during the two world wars, women enjoyed a great deal more freedom as they undertook work previously carried out by men.[22] The increasing autonomy of women meant their relationships were more threatening to the existing fabric of society. Fear of the threat they represented resulted in lesbian women being laughed at and despised.

Christianity considers same-sex relationships sinful. In many countries they are criminal offences. The views of powerful religious and scientific leaders have influenced community thinking to varying degrees at different times and places in history.

In 1882 Western medical science considered lesbianism a congenital disease.[23] In the 1920s, Freud said that homosexuality was an arrested stage of psychosexual development. His complex theories suggested that the 'causes' included unresolved 'oedipal complexes' and castration fears in men, and penis envy in women. Homosexuality was considered by psychiatrists to be a mental illness until 1973, when the American Psychiatric Association removed this diagnosis from its classification of illness. From the 1920s onward, various 'treatments' were employed in an attempt to 'cure' homosexuality. Until the mid-1970s, 'aversion therapy' was used. This involved showing 'patients' pictures of same-sex couples and simultaneously applying either electric shocks or nausea-inducing drugs. The aim was to create a response of aversion rather than attraction, to the same sex.[24] Brain surgery was also used in Australia as a 'cure' for homosexuality up to the early 1970s.[25]

The resurgence of lesbian acceptability began in 1970. In that year, Daughters of Bilitis, Australia's first ever homosexual organisation, was established in Melbourne. It was loosely associated with the American organisation of the same name.[26] Clover, a club for Sydney lesbians, was established in 1972.[27] Throughout the early seventies, lesbian and gay activism forced social change, with many politically focused lesbian groups becoming established.

A Day of International Gay Solidarity was held on 24 June 1978. A march travelled from Taylor Square to Hyde Park in Sydney. Police arrested 53 people. Further confrontation and arrests occurred on 26 June and also in August, when another 104 arrests took place.[28]

The Hyde Park march was the forerunner of what is now the Gay and Lesbian Mardi Gras. On the twentieth anniversary of the march in February 1998, a large contingent of police marched in the Mardi Gras parade carrying a huge banner that read 'We're Here Because We Care'. Messages of support were received from the Premier of New South Wales, the Lord Mayor of Sydney and the Leader of the Federal Opposition. Many politicians, religious, civic and business leaders also marched. It is difficult to imagine anything that has made a greater statement about the changing times!

The intervening twenty years were, however, years of struggle for the individual lesbians whose vision paved the way for change. They formed lesbian support groups, staffed telephone counselling services, ran women's dances, founded newsletters and magazines, wrote books, songs and poetry, organised music festivals and established community centres. Women became academics and conducted research. Artists represented our lives in paint, sculpture, photography and fabric. Lesbians were 'out' in both their private and public sector occupations, and fought for anti-discrimination legislation and change. They bought land and founded lesbian communities. Each and every decision to stand up and be seen was made at personal cost. The struggle was fuelled by lesbians' passion to express their sexuality in the way they chose.

What is women's sexuality?

Sexuality is an 'energy-driven psychological vehicle for pleasure, self-discovery, attachment, and self-esteem'.[29] It has to do with our capacity for desire, arousal and orgasm. It is also about identity. There is a relationship between sexuality and feelings of power and vulnerability. Sexual expression can contribute to our contentment and our capacity for intimacy.[30] Women's sexuality is different from men's. We are different psychologically, hormonally and, obviously, physically.[31] There is a tremendous difference between the things that turn men on and the things that turn women on.[32] We are also different in what satisfies us.[33] Women 'value talking as a way of being close'.[34] Many (but not all) women take pleasure in entwining and embracing. Some women also take pleasure from penetrating and being penetrated.

For women, the goal of sexual activity is not necessarily orgasm. In 1976 Shere Hite reported her findings, after surveying over 2000 women about sex. Hite found that for women, sex is about communication, mutual pleasuring, emotional closeness and body contact.[35] Many women like to touch and caress for the pleasure that it brings, not just as a prelude to orgasm. The majority of women also wanted sex to be part of a mutually respecting relationship, not just for the genital pleasure of climax.[36]

In our culture, doctors, psychiatrists, priests and counsellors are often thought to be the experts on sexuality. Until very recently, most of these 'experts' were male. A great deal of what women believed about themselves was based on the way these authorities said they should behave.[37] Since the 1970s, women, and especially lesbian women, have been redefining their sexuality. They are discovering new ranges of activity, both sexually and in all behaviour patterns and relationships.

MARINA: *Even before I knew I was lesbian I thought my sexual behaviour wasn't right. My boyfriend said I was too aggressive. I used to like to be very active and assertive when we had sex. Jason said it turned him off. I wanted to please him and so I stopped doing it. Later, I was in a relationship with Gina. I would occasionally start to do something*

assertive like getting on top of her, or kissing her passionately.
I would always stop because I was afraid of what she would
think. She told me often that she liked sex with me when I
was 'strong'. It was a long time before I felt safe to be myself
in that way.

If we think that what we feel is not acceptable, we may choose not to acknowledge our true experience. We may hide parts of ourselves. We may not express our wants and needs.

This kind of difficulty creates barriers that prevent us from experiencing our true sexuality. There are other issues that can make it hard to fully engage with our sexual selves. In the rest of this chapter, I am going to talk about the barriers which prevent us from knowing who we are and enjoying our true natures.

Objectification

One aspect of our society's sexual behaviour is objectification. This means treating human beings as if they were objects for the pleasure of another. In recent years there has been opposition to this type of behaviour, but it is still used widely in advertising (a common example is a scantily dressed woman draped over an expensive car). It is found extensively in literature, and is the hallmark of a number of sexual and 'erotic' publications.

As a consequence of being surrounded constantly by these images and messages, many women believe they are (and should be) objects for men's pleasure. As a result, women may try to look and behave in ways they believe will attract men. This has consequences in the way we see ourselves. We feel that our thighs are not shapely enough, our breasts are too small, and our faces are not beautiful. Such negative self-perception has an impact on our self-confidence, our assertiveness in the world and our well-being as a whole. It tends to make us feel powerless rather than powerful. It affects how good we feel sexually.

If a person feels that her body is inadequate she may spend a great deal of emotional and physical energy trying to change it. She will certainly not be spending her time enjoying who she is or finding out more about herself.

If you feel that your body does not reflect your true self then a sense of separation between the mind, emotions, spirit and body may develop.

> **FIONA:** *I felt that I was fat and ugly. But part of me knew that I was beautiful. I felt that there was a being in the middle of me that was beautiful. I used to say, 'I've got a beautiful soul'. I coped by believing that my true soul was somehow separate to my body. I would look at my face in the mirror and think that it was fat. But I would think, 'That's not really me'.*

It can be difficult to wholeheartedly enter a sexual encounter if you don't feel good about yourself. It's even more difficult if there is a sense of separation between your psyche and your body. For some women this sense of disconnection may be profound:

> **JULIE:** *It was difficult for me to stay 'embodied' while I was having sex. I'd had such bad experiences in the past that as soon as I got into bed with someone I would sort of cut off from myself. It felt like it was someone else who was being touched.*

> **CLAIRE:** *I took ages to feel good about my body. When I was in my first lesbian relationship my lover told me again and again that she truly loved my large curves. She told me she found my size and shape a turn-on. Over about a five-year period, I realised my shape was okay. I started wearing sleeveless clothes, shorts, and swimmers. I felt a sense of freedom. For the first time I enjoyed my body. Then I found myself between relationships. I decided I wanted to have a relationship with a man again. One day it hit me with a crunch that I wasn't attractive to men. I didn't fit the stereotype they like. It had an enormous effect on me. The impact on my self-confidence was profound. I went to the hairdressers, I bought make-up and clothes, and went on a*

strict diet. As luck would have it my next relationship was
with my darling Leanne. I still haven't healed the damage I
did to myself during that year when I decided that my body
wasn't okay.

Objectification has some impact on all women. It creates a pressure to conform that affects all of us every day.

If you feel that this issue is affecting you sexually, then simply by noticing that it is happening, you have taken the first step to overcoming the problem. The next step is to start feeling good about your body (see 'Resources').

Stereotypes and sexism

In the past, society has expected that men and women would perform different roles. Women's roles were domestic and passive. Men were the aggressive providers. These stereotypes affected the type of behaviour that was seen as acceptable for women. We were expected to be 'ladylike'. If we were 'tom-boys' our parents and friends made it clear that we were not behaving in a proper manner.

Of course, women were not expected to be assertive sexually. They were to make themselves attractive and wait till they were noticed. They were not expected to enjoy sex. Two hundred years ago one of the hallmarks of a 'lady' was that she did not move whilst having sex.[37] Even today, many young women feel they must not let it be known that they enjoy sex 'too much' or they will quickly be labelled 'slut'.

This conditioning can make it difficult for women to initiate sexual activity. It can also mean that women who do not conform have difficulty being accepted socially. We need to learn how to set these barriers aside before we can enjoy the active, assertive, vibrant parts of our personalities and the strength of our bodies. Sexism has limited our wholehearted enjoyment of sex.

Homophobia and heterosexism

After many years of struggle and courageous action, Australia is beginning to be a more tolerant place for lesbian women to live. There are now anti-discrimination and anti-vilification laws which make it easier to challenge behaviour that discriminates. However, we do not have the same legal rights as heterosexual people (see 'Resources').

In many communities, living as a lesbian still requires courage. Even when straight people don't mean to give offence, they often convey messages that lesbian relationships are not acceptable.

> **KAREN:** *Rachel and I were in a car accident. I was bruised and shaken up but she was badly injured and unconscious. I went with her in the ambulance to the emergency department. I filled out the papers and put myself down as her next of kin. I didn't think twice about it; we've been together for nine years. I always thought her parents accepted me as her life-partner. When Rachel's family arrived at the hospital, her mum took over. The doctors started to accept that she was going to be the decision-maker. I had to insist that I was Rachel's partner and say that I was going to get my solicitor to contact the Anti-Discrimination Board before the doctors started taking me seriously. Later on I found out that I was lucky. If Rachel hadn't regained consciousness and made it very clear that I was her next of kin, I might not have been able to force them to take notice of me.*

> **JUDY:** *My family gets on really well with my lover. It's only with 'little' things that I know they still have a problem. At family gatherings my brother's partner gets introduced as 'This is Dave's wife, Linda'. With us, it's 'This is Judy and her friend Chris.' It makes me feel that they want our relationship hidden. I often wonder how it would be if something happened to one of us. Would they treat it like she was just a friend?*

CHRIS: *Judy's mum is really welcoming, but she's made it clear that she and Dad are embarrassed if Jude and I touch or hold hands. They don't mind at all if her brother gives his wife a big, smoochy kiss.*

Society's attitude to lesbians is often a particular problem when we decide whether or not to tell our parents and families. Straight people don't have to think about it. Our family's reactions give us messages about how they see us.

JUNE: *When my sister got married my family shouted their honeymoon to Cairns and bought them a fridge. When I invited my parents to my commitment ceremony with Jan, Mum said she was sorry she wouldn't be able to come because she would be travelling with Dad on a business trip. They sent a bunch of flowers.*

Not all families are the same.

UNKNOWN WOMAN: *When my younger sister got engaged, my mother bought each of us a beautiful set of cookware. They said they loved us both and wanted to support the life choices that each of us was making by getting us each something for our homes. I felt so affirmed because…I understood they were saying, 'This is your life, and we value you and your choices'.*[38]

LISA: *When I told my family that I was gay they kicked me out. I've lived in a youth refuge for the last two months. My dad won't let me come home unless I give up what he calls my 'immoral lifestyle'.*

In Australia, some lesbian women feel comfortable walking down the street holding hands. Others will kiss their lovers goodbye in the street or at the door. Some of us feel fine about greeting our lovers with a hug in the workplace. However, not all of us do. It depends on the neighbourhood you live in, what your work colleagues are like and how much courage you feel on the day. Only after you have been doing it for a long time do these things come naturally.

Despite laws designed to protect us, I have friends who have had to move house because of anti-lesbian violence and abuse from their neighbours. If a lesbian decides to be 'out' in her workplace, it can be a real risk. Some women still choose not to come out; they simply avoid talking about their personal lives.

When women decide to be open, there are decisions to be made constantly, reinforcing the message that you are different from most of the people around you. If you happen to mention your partner in casual conversation you will often be met with responses like 'What does he do?' On each and every occasion, you have to decide whether to correct the wrong assumption. Living as a lesbian requires courage. Being an out lesbian requires true strength of character.

The most profound impact comes from internalised homophobia. This is what happens when we have deeply absorbed the message that what we are is not alright. Internalised homophobia is the name for feeling wrong, guilty, immoral, dirty, or in any way not acceptable because of being lesbian.

If we are afraid of what our friends and workmates think, we may be withdrawn. Some women feel compelled to hide their lives. Others have lied, inventing fictitious boyfriends, husbands and families. Hiding, or living a lie, means that it is difficult to relate with openness to co-workers in other matters. You never know when the conversation may turn to something where you have to be on your guard.

When at a deep level you have absorbed the message that you are different, and unacceptable, it affects your self-esteem. This can result in negative feelings about having sex. It can also make it very difficult to meet partners and other lesbian women. If a heterosexual woman decides she wants a new relationship, any man who is unattached is part of a pool of potential candidates. All she has to do is work out if he is interested. There are established rituals for making contact. Lesbian women first of all have to work out who, among all the women they come in contact with, might be interested in a same-sex relationship. (See Chapter 11 for more about this.)

JOAN: *When I first came out it was awful. I knew I was gay, but I didn't know how to find any other gay women. I'd sit on the train 'dyke-spotting' and try to work up the courage to say 'hello' if I thought a woman looked like she might be a dyke. I never did. I was too afraid that I'd be wrong. Once two women came to talk to my tech class. They were both in their sixties and said that they'd been companions for many years. They both had short hair and looked butch. They were very familiar with each other. I thought they were a couple. I went up after the class, introduced myself, said I was gay and asked some sort of leading question (I can't remember what). They were both horrified. To this day I still think they were dykes. But I learned my lesson. I was never that up-front again.*

It can be difficult to actually ask a woman out. If you have previously been in heterosexual relationships you may be used to men taking the initiative. It can be very nerve-racking to pick the phone up and actually ask a woman out on a date. Don't despair, though, it gets easier with practice.

Sexual abuse

Any woman who has been sexually abused may experience barriers to fully and joyfully experiencing her sexuality. Unfortunately, 'sexual aggression against women is pervasive in our society'.[39] Studies suggest that one-quarter of girls are victims of sexual abuse while still under the age of eighteen years.[40] More than forty-four per cent of women experience forced physical sexual contact at some point in their lives.[41] Much higher numbers of women experience sexual abuse, which falls short of physical assault.[42]

Sexual abuse is a spectrum that includes violent rape, incest, 'date rape' and unwanted sexual touching. Sexually based name calling, unwelcome sexual jokes and the unwanted wolf-whistle in the street are examples of sexual harassment. All of these acts involve objectification. One human person sees another human being as an object for sexual pleasure. Such abuse always involves a misuse of power.

All of these abuses involve violation of either the physical or the psychic self. Women who have been violated may face difficulties that are a consequence of being abused. Some women who have been sexually abused need to take a break from sex altogether until they feel ready to enjoy it again. If you have been a victim of sexual abuse and you feel it is affecting your present relationships and sexual activity, you are not alone. If you have been sexually assaulted, seek counselling. Seek out self-help groups. Look at the list of resources in the back of this book. Talking to other women about what happened can also help.

Coming through it all

Sexism, objectification, homophobia and sexual abuse have touched every woman. Despite this, vast numbers of women live healthy and fulfilled lives. However, some women have been so wounded that emotional and physical survival is difficult. Most of us have been deeply affected by one or other of these cultural phenomena. In order to be able to get into bed and make love wholeheartedly with another human being, many of us have needed to heal the damage first.

The very first step towards healing is acknowledging the impact. The next step is protecting yourself from further harm. Notice if those around you have an impact on you in a sexist, homophobic or abusive way, and act to prevent harm to yourself (and others). Another important factor is to notice every time your present behaviour may be influenced by what happened in the past. The key is to always be gentle with yourself: give yourself time, don't judge yourself harshly, never push yourself to change quickly. Both lesbian and heterosexual women face these issues. There are positive things that may be discovered on the journey towards healing. Some of us would never have known about our strength of spirit if we had not travelled through the black shadows of our abusive past. We learned that we have capacities we never imagined and that the human spirit is greater than we knew. We have learned about the path towards wholeness. Our journeys have made us who we are.

Life being what it is, the path is a spiral one. You may think you have healed the wounds, but find that thoughts and feelings surface sometimes. They may be triggered by something in the present or they may simply arise, seemingly of their own volition. New abusive situations may occur. If you find yourself in a raw or tender state, nurture yourself; give yourself the gift of space and time to know your feelings. If necessary, seek out a counsellor. Discover the value of support groups.

As our wounds mend, we move towards connection with our inner selves as well as with others. The move towards personal wholeness and integrity also allows us to enjoy the sex life of our choice.

2

Knowing Your Own Body

Most girls have grown into women with very little idea of what their genital area looks like. Many were given strong messages that their genitals were taboo. Very few of us have sat down with a mirror to find out what we look like 'down there'. Even fewer women have explored their own smell and taste.

Lesbians have the privilege of becoming intimate with other women's bodies. However, we may not necessarily understand how they work. We may see our sexual parts without knowing much about how they function. We may know the proper names for our anatomy and yet choose to use other words.

> **LIZ:** *It's about reclaiming our parts as really wonderful gorgeous, sensual bits, rather than having somebody else describe them for us in cold medical language.*

In this chapter I will use the medical words that describe women's bodies. However, if there are other words that are used by lesbian women, I will use these also.

Feminist women's groups have done ground-breaking work to encourage people to get to know themselves. They have produced classic books such as *Our Bodies Ourselves*[1] and *A New View of a Woman's Body*[2] and formed self-help groups which aim to teach women about their own anatomy and health.

> In the 1980s, I was involved in a Women's Health Centre. A woman wanted to run a course called 'Women's Bodies'. Approval was given by the board to go ahead.
>
> Someone asked, 'Are you going to do the course, Carol?'
>
> 'Me?' I was astonished. Why would I want to do a course called 'Women's Bodies'?. I thought that I knew everything there was to know about women's bodies – I owned one, wasn't that enough? To my utter amazement, the course involved looking at our own bodies. The teachers encouraged us to go home with mirrors, speculums, lights and our friends and find out what we actually looked like. We learned about our genitals, breasts and breast checks and how to care for our sexual health.

So what is there to know?

EROGENOUS ZONES

These are parts of the body where stimulation gives rise to sexual desire or excitement.

In traditional medical teaching, the erogenous zones are the:

- breasts;
- genitals;
- anus and rectum.

However, they can also include lips, ears, back of neck, toes, inner thighs and lower back. In fact, the whole skin may be treated as an erogenous zone!

There is another extremely important erogenous zone. I feel compelled to give credit to the person who told me about it. When I was in medical school, we had a lecture on sexuality given by a gentleman who came into our lecture theatre in a wheelchair. As a result of a car accident, he was paralysed, and had no sensation from his shoulders down. He spoke about the ways in which he was able to give pleasure to his wife and the sexual satisfaction that they both received from it. He said, 'Never forget, the most important erogenous zone lies between your ears. It is your mind'.

Breasts

> **RHONDA:** *I can have an orgasm just from having my nipples squeezed or sucked. It seems like it's a direct line to my clitoris.*

> **TONI:** *I used to hate my breasts. They were so big they gave me neckache and backache. I always felt that men were looking at them. The best thing I ever did was get them 'reduced'. I've never really had much pleasure from Rachel stroking or sucking them, but she likes to, so I let her.*

> **LOUISE:** *Just looking at women's breasts turns me on. I love to watch my partner get dressed. It is all I can do to keep my hands off her.*

Breasts come in a spectacular array of sizes and shapes. For some women, the whole breast is an erogenous zone. For others, the nipple is exquisitely sensitive. However, some women do not like having their breasts touched at all.

Breasts may have been altered by surgery for cancer, or for cosmetic reasons. Scarring may affect sensation and the way women feel about their breasts.

Internally, breasts are composed of fifteen to twenty lobes or sections, which are separated by fatty tissue. The lobes are comprised of lobules that contain milk-secreting cells. The milk collects in ducts, ca, mammary ducts. Ligaments support the breasts. The amount of fatty tissue and the suspensory ligaments determine the shape of the breasts.

The mammary ducts (shown in Figure 1 below) come to the surface at the nipple, which is comprised of erectile tissue. This allows the nipple to become stiff and hard when you are aroused or cold. Inverted nipples do not stand up. They are a variation of normal.

To look at, the breast swells off the chest wall, and there is a nipple that is surrounded by an area called the areola. If the woman has been pregnant, her areola will have become darker in colour about eight weeks after she conceived. It then usually remains a darker shade for the rest of her life.

Genitals

One of the easiest ways to become familiar with your genitals is to have a look. Get out a mirror, a light, find a quiet space and investigate. You will be following in the footsteps of the women who showed the world the truth about women's anatomy.

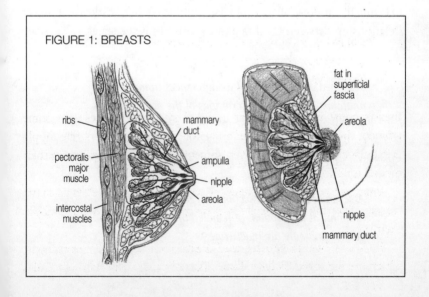

FIGURE 1: BREASTS

ribs

mammary duct

pectoralis major muscle

ampulla

nipple

intercostal muscles

areola

fat in superficial fascia

areola

nipple

mammary duct

...am' of the Federation of Feminist Women's Health ...rica was comprised of ordinary women. In 1981 their ...iew of *A Woman's Body* was published. In it they state ... our pants and compared ourselves with illustrations in the mo... ...pected anatomy texts, both American and European'.[3] They concluded that the anatomy taught to medical students was simply wrong.

> *Most medical illustrators are men – which explains why*
> *there have been intricate cross-sections of the penis since*
> *Leonardo da Vinci's time, while comparable drawings of the*
> *female organs often have areas of empty space. Distortions*
> *can be seen in almost any drawing. For example, the vagina*
> *is almost always shown as a gaping hole or an open tunnel,*
> *which it is not.*

These women were able to show that the clitoris was much more extensive and important to female sexual satisfaction than had previously been believed.

Despite the fact that medical knowledge of anatomy was shown to be deficient, very little changed until 1998. In that year, Dr Helen O'Connell, an Australian urologist, published her work 'Anatomical Relationship Between Urethra and Clitoris'. In it she states:

> *Typically, the human female perineal anatomy is briefly*
> *described only in terms of its differences from the male...*
> *anatomy. Frequently, descriptions of the neurovascular*
> *supply...are scant or absent.*[4]

She concluded:

> *A series of detailed dissections suggest that current*
> *anatomical descriptions of female human urethral and*
> *genital anatomy are inaccurate.*[5]

You can be the authority on your own anatomy. If you sit with a mirror between your legs and a good light shining on it you will see your vulva. The vulva includes the fatty pubic mound (also called 'the mons pubis'), the outer lips of the vagina, the inner lips of the vagina, the clitoris, the vestibule of the vagina, and the perineum (which is the area between the anus and the vagina).

Moving from outside to inside you will first come across the outer lips of the vagina, which are also called the labia majora. The outer lips usually have some pubic hair on them and are comprised of fat. The round ligament, which runs from the uterus (or womb), has branches that end in the fat of the pubic mound.[6]

If you part the outer lips you will come across the inner lips (the labia minora). The inner lips are often a deeper colour than the outer lips. They may range in colour from deep pink or red to dark brown or black. Like the areola of the breast, the inner lips usually become a darker shade when a woman is about eight weeks pregnant. They are usually thinner than the outer lips and are soft and velvety to touch. They vary greatly in size and shape from woman to woman. In many women the inner lips are longer than the outer lips. One side can be larger than the other.

The inner lips join at the top, to form the hood (or prepuce) of the clitoris. One or two folds of skin usually meet under or at the clitoris and are called the frenulum (see Fig. 3).

The most well-known part of the clitoris (the glans clitoris) is located near where the inner lips of the vagina meet. In the past the clitoris has been described as a 'little button'. Since the work done by the Federation of Feminist Women's Health Centers, we have known that it is much more extensive than that. Dr Helen O'Connell's recent dissections have confirmed this.[7]

The clitoris contains erectile tissue, which becomes filled with blood when you are sexually excited. It is comprised not only of the glans (the 'button' which you may know from masturbation or sex play), but also the shaft (which can be felt in many women when it becomes erect), two crura or legs and the bulb of the clitoris.

The glans, which is the part you can see, varies in size from woman to woman. It also varies in shape, colour and sensitivity.

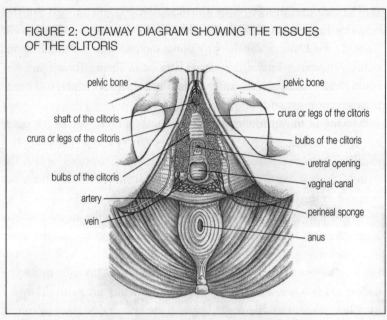

FIGURE 2: CUTAWAY DIAGRAM SHOWING THE TISSUES OF THE CLITORIS

pelvic bone
pelvic bone
shaft of the clitoris
crura or legs of the clitoris
crura or legs of the clitoris
bulbs of the clitoris
uretral opening
bulbs of the clitoris
vaginal canal
artery
perineal sponge
vein
anus

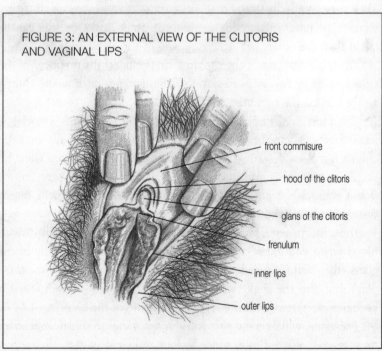

FIGURE 3: AN EXTERNAL VIEW OF THE CLITORIS AND VAGINAL LIPS

front commisure
hood of the clitoris
glans of the clitoris
frenulum
inner lips
outer lips

The crura or legs flare out from the base of the shaft, and extend deep within the pelvic area along each side of the pubic bones. The bulb is a mass of erectile spongy tissue surrounding the urethra, and running down both sides of the urethra and the vaginal opening. It is believed that there is also erectile tissue between the vagina and anus. In sexual excitement the legs and bulb of the clitoris are squeezed and stimulated by movement of the pelvic floor muscles.

Ligaments extend from a broad base within the mons and connect to the body of the clitoris and also into the labia majora.[8] The fact is that the clitoris actually extends on both sides round the vagina. It is intrinsically connected to the pubis, the labia majora and the perineum. This may explain why stimulation in these areas can cause clitoral sensations and orgasm.

Vagina is the word used to describe the space (or potential space) which leads from outside the body to the uterus or womb. Normally the vagina lies flat and closed. It has strong muscular walls. It is also sometimes called 'the birth canal'. In sexual excitement it may balloon into a large space and, for some women, accommodate a lover's whole fist. It is big enough, of course, to accommodate a baby's journey to the outside world.

Many women enjoy the sensation of something inside them (for example, a finger or two, or a dildo), but some women do not like the idea or feeling of vaginal penetration. If you are not relaxed, or have previously been a victim of sexual or other trauma, the vaginal walls may be tense. It may be painful to have anything inserted. What goes into your vagina must always be of your choice.

Contraction of vaginal muscles that causes pain is called vaginismus. Some women may suffer from this and also have happy lesbian sex lives, without any desire or need for change. Others would like to enjoy penetration. If vaginismus gets in the way of your sexual enjoyment, see p. 118.

About an inch inside the opening to the vagina, there may be a ring of tissue called the hymen. In women who wear tampons, are sexually active or play sport, the hymen will usually have been torn, leaving only remnants. In women who have been sexually active for some time, or who have had children there may be only a few tags of skin left,

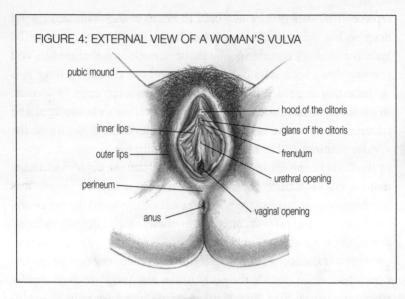

FIGURE 4: EXTERNAL VIEW OF A WOMAN'S VULVA

pubic mound

hood of the clitoris

inner lips

glans of the clitoris

outer lips

frenulum

urethral opening

perineum

anus

vaginal opening

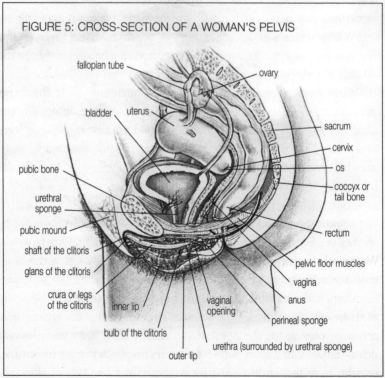

FIGURE 5: CROSS-SECTION OF A WOMAN'S PELVIS

fallopian tube

ovary

bladder

uterus

sacrum

cervix

pubic bone

os

coccyx or tail bone

urethral sponge

pubic mound

rectum

shaft of the clitoris

glans of the clitoris

pelvic floor muscles

vagina

crura or legs of the clitoris

anus

inner lip

vaginal opening

bulb of the clitoris

perineal sponge

outer lip

urethra (surrounded by urethral sponge)

representing where the hymen used to be. In women who have never been sexually active, the hymen may be a membrane of skin with an aperture that varies from a pinpoint in size to one which may admit one or two fingers.

Between the glans clitoris and the vagina is the urethra or opening to the bladder. The urethra may be small and difficult to see. It can be extremely close to the vagina and is sometimes located just inside the vaginal opening.

The urethra is the tube that carries urine from the bladder when we urinate. The Federation of Feminist Women's Health Centres describes the urethra as being wrapped in the paraurethral sponge.[9] This is a dense mass of blood vessels and spongy tissue. The thickest part of the paraurethral sponge lies between the urethra and the upper vaginal wall. Dr O'Connell's dissections have confirmed that except where the vaginal wall is adjacent, the urethra is 'surrounded by erectile tissue in all directions'.[10] Within the sponge is the paraurethral gland.

Stimulation of this area can be very exciting. Some women report that during sexual stimulation, particularly of this area, a large amount of clear fluid is emitted. Some call this 'female ejaculation'. Since the 1920s, doctors have argued about the nature of this fluid. Some assert that it is 'ejaculate', similar in nature to that produced by men (without the sperm), believing it is produced in the glands that surround the urethra. Others insist that it is urine. Many doctors have ridiculed the idea of female ejaculation. They state that urine is released as a result of 'stress incontinence'. However, women who experience this release and have no other problems with incontinence note that it is pleasurable.

JAN: *It smells different! It tastes different!*

Women also report that the fluid does not stain bed sheets in the same way. It is released in gushes at orgasm. It therefore does not have any function related to lubrication.

This argument has not yet been settled. The nature of the fluid has not been proven but it doesn't really matter if its ejaculate or urine. What is important is to realise that releasing an amount of fluid at orgasm is healthy, normal, and not at all uncommon.

The place on the front of the vaginal wall where you can stimulate the paraurethral sponge is known as the 'G spot' or 'Grafenburg spot'.[11]

The fluid which some women say is released when their G spot is stimulated is clear. It may range in quantity from a few drops to a large amount. Women report multiple orgasms from this stimulation. The strength and tone of a woman's pubococcygeus muscle influences her ability to orgasm from stimulation within the vagina.

> **JILL:** *It blew me away the first time Heather and I discovered my G spot. I thought I was pissing myself. When we read up on it later we found it was ejaculate.*

If you have never found your G spot and would like to, or would like to learn how to strengthen your pubococcygeus muscles, see 'Applied Anatomy' (Appendix 2).

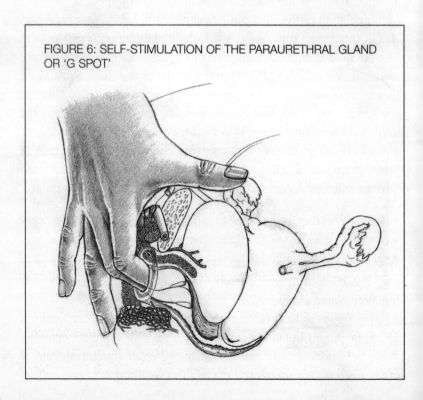

FIGURE 6: SELF-STIMULATION OF THE PARAURETHRAL GLAND OR 'G SPOT'

There is another area, deep within the vagina, where stimulation causes pleasure. This is the perineal sponge. It is located deep to the back wall of the vagina, approximately opposite the 'G spot', and lies between the vagina and the perineum. There are two sets of glands located on each side of the opening to the vagina. The larger pair is located on each side of the vaginal opening and is most commonly called 'Bartholin's glands'. These do secrete a few drops of fluid during sexual arousal. There are also several smaller glands, on each side of the opening of the vagina, called the 'lesser vestibular glands'. Their function is unknown. Women are only usually aware of these glands if they become infected and swollen.

About eight to ten centimetres inside your vagina lies the cervix, which is the mouth of the womb (or uterus). When you feel deep inside your vagina you will touch the cervix, which feels firm. It was once thought that the cervix did not cause any sexual sensation. However, it is now believed that it can contribute to vaginal sensations that lead to orgasm, and that the cervix may spasm at the time of orgasm. You can look at your cervix with a light, a mirror and a disposable speculum.[12]

The anus and rectum

The anus is the entrance to the rectum, which is at the end of the large bowel. The anus is about two centimetres long and has two rings of strong muscle called the internal and external sphincters. It opens into the rectum, which is where faeces is stored until defecation. Like the vagina, the rectum is capable of expanding to quite a large space. Some women like the feeling of rectal penetration. This can be done with fingers, dildos, fists, enemas or other objects.

The external anal sphincter can be relaxed voluntarily. Movement of the inner sphincter is usually involuntary. Before anal penetration can comfortably occur, the inner sphincter needs to be relaxed. This can occur with sexual excitement. If you attempt to penetrate the anus when both sphincters are not relaxed, it is likely to be painful and may cause tearing. However, if you are excited by anal sex it is possible to learn to relax both sphincters at will. For more information about anal sex, see p.48.

Haemorrhoids are varicose veins that occur just inside the anus. They may prolapse so that they come out of the anus. Anal fissures are cracks in the tissue. They may become infected and possibly bleed. Both of these conditions can make anal penetration painful. If you or your partner have these problems, you may find other types of sexual stimulation more pleasurable.

SEXUAL RESPONSE

Masters and Johnson, pioneering researchers in the field of human sexuality, were the first to describe the way sexual response cycles work. They outlined four phases.

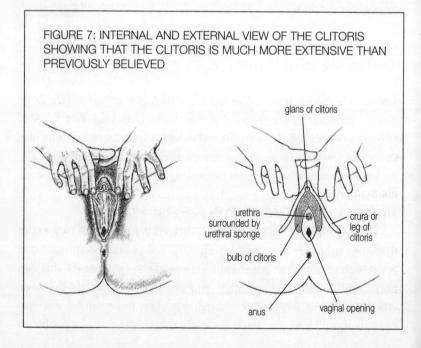

FIGURE 7: INTERNAL AND EXTERNAL VIEW OF THE CLITORIS SHOWING THAT THE CLITORIS IS MUCH MORE EXTENSIVE THAN PREVIOUSLY BELIEVED

glans of clitoris

urethra surrounded by urethral sponge

crura or leg of clitoris

bulb of clitoris

anus

vaginal opening

Excitement

Erotic stimulus, sights, smells, sounds, thoughts and touch can cause the glans of the clitoris to swell. The shaft may start to become erect as the whole organ becomes engorged with blood. The vagina 'sweats' lubricant. The genitals get warmer and swell. The breasts swell and the nipples may start to become erect. There is also an increase in pulse rate and blood pressure.

Plateau

The genital tissues become even more filled with blood. The inner lips may change colour and become markedly darker. The hood of the clitoris may enlarge and pull on the shaft. The perineal sponge thickens and fills with blood. The uterus, tubes and ovaries swell. Women may have begun rhythmic movements. Breasts may have increased in size by up to one quarter. The nipples become erect. The entrance to the vagina may tighten and the back portion may balloon into a cavity.

Orgasm

When the sensations have reached maximum intensity, strong rhythmic muscle contractions occur. The clitoris shortens and tucks in under its hood. Some women experience spasms in their hands or feet. Breaths become faster and the heart rate increases. The pulse rate also increases. There may be widespread tingling sensation felt all over the body. The clitoris and vagina may rhythmically contract. The anal sphincter may contract. Women perspire and their skin may become flushed. Masters and Johnson believed that orgasm was the reason why people have sex.

Resolution

The body relaxes and returns to its pre-excitement state.

This description of the sexual response cycle gave our culture a very useful starting point in understanding sexuality. Helen Kaplan[13] took our understanding a step forward. She described a cycle similar to that proposed by Masters and Johnson. However, she suggested that 'Desire' was the first stage in the cycle.

JoAnn Loulan has developed an even more precise model of women's sexual responses.[14] It is set out in the diagram below. Loulan states that the goal of sexual activity is pleasure. She believes that you can experience pleasure without any other previous stage except willingness. All of the other states may be bypassed. Her view of the sexual response cycle accurately represents the experience of many women. She sets out her stages as follows:

Stage 1 – Willingness
This is the decision to be sexually intimate. It does not matter why you have decided to be physically sexual. It doesn't even matter if you don't particularly want to have sex. You are just willing to. You may want to be sexual because it creates intimacy, because you want to build a more fulfilling sex life, because you think you'll probably enjoy it once you get into it, whatever. However, the willingness must not be of the 'Oh, well, she wants it so I'll put up with it' variety. Rather, it is a conscious decision, even if you don't have a great deal of desire at the time. This stage may lead to some or all of the other stages. It may lead simply to pleasure. Or it can lead to shutdown and back to the resting state.

Stage 2 – Desire
According to Loulan, this is 'wanting to have sex because it feels good and you're attracted to someone'.[15] Desire may be intellectual; that is, experienced in our minds. It may be emotional, when you have strong feelings about a woman and want to have sex with her because of those feelings. Desire may also be physical, marked by the strong stirrings of lust that we feel. This stage can also lead to excitement, shutdown, resting, or pleasure.

Stage 3, 4 and 5 are Excitement, Engorgement and Orgasm.
These are similar to the stages described by Masters and Johnston.

Stage 6 – Pleasure
Loulan asserts: 'Pleasure is the purpose of sexuality'. She goes on to say that it is possible to experience any of the above stages, and experience

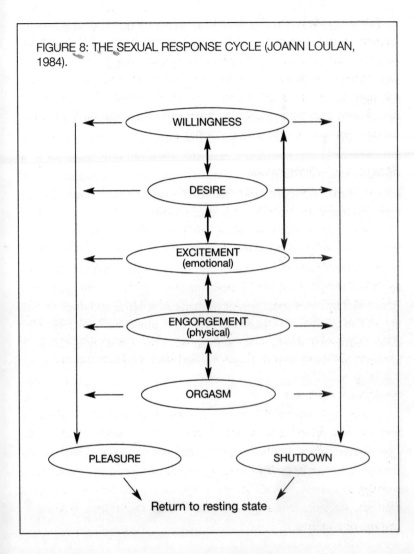

FIGURE 8: THE SEXUAL RESPONSE CYCLE (JOANN LOULAN, 1984).

pleasure. Neither orgasm, nor any other stage, is required to feel pleasure. You can get pleasure just from the fact that you were willing to have a sexual experience, even if you shut down quickly after starting. She has an expanded definition of pleasure, which depends on what the woman likes and wants.

Loulan notes that it is also possible to go through all the above stages and not experience pleasure.

The stages do not necessarily follow one after the other and may be mixed up. You may go straight from any stage to any other stage. For instance, you may quickly go from willingness to orgasm.

Shutdown

This can happen at any time in the cycle. It may be due to fatigue, anxiety, depression, disinterest, distraction, anger, fear of sex or intimacy, or stress. Shutdown may also be a physical response to a stimulus that you find unpleasant. It may lead away from sexual activity to the resting state or some other physical or emotional state. It may also lead back into further sexual activity.

Loulan argues that her more complex sexual response cycle is 'much truer to women's sexual experience'. I have not conducted a multi-centre, randomised, double-blind, controlled trial to verify her assertion. My personal and clinical impressions are that she is correct. Her model includes space for all women's experience and does not set up orgasm as a goal for 'good sex'. Her new model explains a broader range of the sexual cycle. 'No woman has to feel that she is different because her experience doesn't match the Masters and Johnson paradigm.'[16]

3

Knowing Another Woman's Body

Before you decide that you want to become intimate with other women, there are a few issues you may want to think about. Some women decide they want to know other women's bodies because they have actively chosen (or are considering) a lesbian lifestyle. Others find themselves wanting physical closeness with other women without making such a choice. We often interact with each other intimately, but non-sexually. Sometimes we have very intimate friendships with other women. There may be an intense emotional connection. This may become an easy physical familiarity and we may know each other's bodies well. And yet, if there is no genital intimacy we may consider that these relationships are non-sexual.

In 1980 Adrienne Rich expanded the definition of lesbianism to include the 'lesbian continuum' which she described as

> *A range – through each woman's life, and throughout history – of woman-identified experience; not simply...genital sexual experience.*[1]

Rich considered the possibility

> *That all women – from the infant suckling her mother's*
> *breast, to the grown woman experiencing orgasmic sensations*
> *while suckling her own child…; to two women, like Virginia*
> *Woolf's Chloe and Olivia, who share a laboratory; to the*
> *woman dying at ninety, touched and handled by women –*
> *exist on a lesbian continuum, we can see ourselves as moving*
> *in and out of this continuum, whether we identify ourselves*
> *as lesbian or not.*[2]

Many women know other woman's bodies non-sexually. Large numbers of us work in caring professions – we look after the hygiene and physical needs of others. At home, we are usually the ones who bath and care for the very young and the very old. Some of us like to swim in secluded places with no clothes, some like to spa and bath together. We share the locker rooms of gyms and work places. Some of us enjoy the absence of clothes, and feel that being around unclothed women is an intimacy and a privilege.

One of the things that can happen through being around unclothed women is that you become more comfortable with yourself, especially if you are with women who are comfortable with their bodies. When you see women without clothes you notice that we come in all shapes and sizes. You realise that big women, skinny women, lumpy women and women with illness and injury are all beautiful women. The belief perpetuated by the media, that beauty is a size 10 eighteen-year-old, has to be recognised for what it is – a myth.

Deciding that you want to know another woman's body sexually is a major step. It may be a single casual encounter, or a lifestyle choice that has been pushing its way into your heart and mind for some time.

For some women, the first experience with a woman can be very frightening. Others say that they were totally at ease.

> **MELANIE:** *I knew that I was probably lesbian. Even though I*
> *went out with men, I'd been thinking about sex with women*
> *since I was fifteen. My first time with a woman was when I*

*was twenty-three. I worked in welfare and she was my
supervisor. From the first time I set eyes on her there was
electricity between us. She was eight years older than me,
and a very experienced dyke. I would hang onto every word
she said. I would make excuses to be in her presence.
Because of our work we didn't do anything about it. When I
left the placement she asked me out to dinner. I knew as I
said 'yes' to dinner that I was hoping we would end up in
bed. I was absolutely terrified, but I was like a moth to a
flame. I wanted her. But I didn't really want to think that I
might be a lesbian, and all that would mean. I was also
terrified of the sex. I thought I wouldn't know what to do. She
was incredibly gentle and wonderful. It worked out fine.*

ZOE: *It amazed me how easy and natural the first time was.
Neither of us had been with a woman before, but we both
just slipped into it. Like breathing.*

For me to have sex with anyone, I have to like and respect them. In
letting them touch me, and go inside my body, I also let them touch my
spirit, heart and mind. I let them know me very deeply. I have learned
over the years that I am unable to have sex without a relationship.
For some women, a sexual relationship has a strongly spiritual
meaning.

LOU: *Nita and I are soul mates. Our sex life is part of our
connection with each other. When we make love, all our
barriers go down. Lying in her arms is bliss.*

Not everyone is the same. Women also delight in the absolute physical
enjoyment of sex.

GERALDINE: *Respect them, be buggered. I just want to bonk
with them. I don't care if I never see them again.*

> **JAC:** *Gee, I think I can remember the names of every woman I've slept with – at least their first names anyway.*

The capacity of women to predict the desires and feelings of other women is called gender empathy. Not all lesbian couples experience it. Women with diverse backgrounds may not foresee each other's needs and wants. However, some couples find that they anticipate each other's wishes emotions and even thoughts.

> **GINA:** *I couldn't believe how easy it was when I started going to bed with Marina. I had been divorced two years and I didn't think I wanted another relationship with anyone. Sex was not something my husband had asked for. It was something he demanded. If I didn't 'come across' I got a hard time verbally and cold shoulder treatment until I did. My satisfaction or pleasure was never in his mind. Sex became just a duty. So a sexual relationship was not something I was considering. Marina and I decided to do a massage course together. We swapped massages at home. One day after I gave her a massage we ended up kissing. We were both single and there didn't seem to be any reason why we shouldn't go to bed, so we did. It was so gentle and easy. She seemed to know what I wanted. She could sense, without me telling her, that I wanted to go slow.*

Women may be surprised at how different they are physically.

> **SAM:** *I've had three children. It's easy for Fiona to fit her whole fist inside me and I love it. She's never had children. Her vagina is so small and tight I worry about hurting her. I've still got a lot to learn about her body before I feel comfortable.*

There may be practical barriers to getting close to women sexually. Some women need to get used to the smells and tastes of women. Others are particular about cleanliness.

NINA: *I don't like having oral sex unless I know Leanne has had a shower. She doesn't mind whether I've had one or not. She says she likes the smell of me and she says she likes it as much if I smell strong. She says it's just different. She loves oral sex anyway. I'm not always that comfortable letting her lick me if I know I smell strongly or I've got my period.*

We often find it difficult to ask for what we want sexually. We have been conditioned to be passive sexually. Women are programmed to look after the needs of others rather than to seek to have their own desires met.

CLAIRE: *Even though I'm an intelligent, assertive woman, I sometimes find it difficult to actually say what I want in bed. Sometimes I'm embarrassed about what I'd like. But other times I simply don't know why I can't open my mouth and get the words out.*

With all of these issues it is important to work out how you feel, and to go for what you want. If you would like to try oral sex, but only if the other person has showered, ask for that. You might find that once you get used to the smells and tastes of a showered woman the different odours and flavours of an unshowered one could turn you on. If you are setting out on the adventure of interacting with women sexually, there will be a whole range of new experiences ahead. As with all sexual activity, it will be easier if you make sure the physical environment is comfortable for you. This could involve attending to relatively simple matters. If you feel the cold, it may be important to have a warm room. In winter this can take a bit of planning but it will be worth it if you intend to have a relaxed sexual encounter.

It is also essential to be able to communicate with your partner about what you want and like. The following chapters address these issues.

4

What Do Lesbians Do?

t seems that there is a mystery about what lesbian sexual activity involves. To some heterosexual people, lesbian sex is not seen as real sex. In fact, sexual activity between a woman and a man is not regarded as 'real sex' unless the penis ends up in the vagina. Anything else is 'not going all the way' or is 'just foreplay' or 'mucking around'. These views are widespread. They make it difficult to imagine that a wide variety of other activities could be very satisfying.

> **SHEREE:** *I finally told a friend at work that my 'flatmate' was really my lover. Since then she has asked me about how my family 'cope' and about lesbian nightclubs and concerts and all sorts of different things about what it's like to be a lesbian. She seemed really interested in lesbian life. One day she said, 'What do you actually DO?' I couldn't believe she had no idea. I didn't know how to answer her. Maybe she thinks we stand on our heads naked.*

Lesbian tradition has it that when Queen Victoria was asked to sign legislation making homosexual activity a criminal offence in England, she sniffed, deleted the paragraphs relating to women, and commented that she could imagine nothing interesting that women might do together. She then endorsed the law prohibiting male homosexual behaviour.

> **CATH:** *When I was deciding that I was sexually attracted to women I thought I knew what they did together, although I kept having doubts. I wondered if there was something else I hadn't thought of.*

One of the things lesbians don't do a great deal of is to talk explicitly about their sexual activity. This is probably because we are normal members of our society, and generally in our culture, we don't discuss who puts what bits where in bed. This has added to the mystery surrounding lesbian sex. Really it isn't a mystery. Lesbian lovemaking often takes more time than heterosexual sex. Its aim may often be closeness rather than orgasm.[2] However, lesbians are more likely to have multiple orgasms than their straight sisters.[3]

Every possible sexual activity (including the heterosexual 'missionary position' with the man on top and woman underneath) has at some time in history been judged to be either sinful, amoral, unsanitary or in some way not acceptable. Human beings love to judge the sexual behaviour of others. The lesbian community at times falls into this trap. Some lesbians believe that celibate lesbians aren't really lesbian. Some think that sadomasochism is 'too violent'. Others feel that 'vanilla sex'[4] is 'limited, boring or repetitive... increasingly disparaged...'[5] These activities are described and discussed later in this chapter.

JoAnn Loulan has observed that some people think that lesbians have to have sex in a particular way to be lesbians. 'Nonsense! Lesbian sex is anything two lesbians do together. Monitoring our own and other's sexual behaviour is in no-one's interest but our oppressors.'[6]

Sexual activity between adults and children, and sex that is non-consenting or coercive, is against the law. It is a mark of our civilisation's maturity that we now take real steps to protect the vulnerable. However, provided we are adult and capable of true consent, the way we have sex is no-one's business but our own. If we are critical of the way others choose to express their sexuality, then we create damage in the same way as those who discriminate against homosexual people and other minority groups. Thankfully, our civilisation is moving towards an acceptance of diversity that permits each of us to be who we are.

Many lesbians are uncomfortable with some of the activities in this chapter. That is okay. It is important that every woman is at ease with the way she chooses to express herself sexually. Whether you do, or do not do, any of these activities does not mean a thing about how satisfying and fulfilling your sexual activity is.

My experience, and what women have told me, limits my descriptions of what lesbians do. The activities I set out are not a complete list. If there is something you feel I should have written about, please contact me. Most lesbians will do some but not all of the activities I describe.

Talking

For many women, sex is about contact. Talking is a way to initiate contact. It can be a path to connection of the mind, emotions, spirit and soul. Talking often helps us ease into touching.

> **LOU:** *Talking is as important to me as anything else we do in bed. We will be snuggled up together chatting, cuddling and being sensual. We can kiss for hours. Just mouths. Touching and licking and sucking. We might sort of just sort of slide into being more sexual. If we didn't talk, I wouldn't want to have sexual intimacy. I'm making love to a person, not just a body. Sometimes we'll be making love, stop and talk and then drift back to making love (or off to sleep, depending on our*

mood). It's like a dance, weaving in out of sensual, sexual space.

GINA: *I love it when Marina talks to me in bed. Her moans let me know if what I'm doing is working. I love it when she tells me what she wants. It makes me more aroused that she can be so explicit.*

Talking can have an extremely erotic dimension.

HEATHER: *Before we started a relationship, Jill was outrageous. She had a very clear picture of what she wanted. She used words like other people use erotic touch. I remember distinctly what she said the evening we first made love: She took my hand and said something like: 'Heather, I would love to slowly undress you. I'd start by very gently unbuttoning your blouse. Then I'd run my fingers tips from your ears down to your neck. I'd lightly brush along your collarbones and slowly, soft as a whisper start to stroke your cleavage. If it felt okay to you, I'd softly brush all the surfaces of your breasts. I'd slowly tease the areas around your nipples…' She went on telling me what she'd do all the way down my body. She was very graphic. I was an absolute mess listening to her. She didn't have to try very hard to persuade me.*

Giving or receiving a graphic description of what might be about to take place can be very erotic.

Talking also has a vitally important place in our sex lives; in new relationships, we must assess the risk of contracting sexually transmitted infections and negotiate safe sex. Talking to each other is the only way to do this. Chapter 5 gives more information about negotiating safe sex.

Touching

Sex is about touching in the most intimate of all ways. Touching is often where it all starts. For women who are strongly attracted to each other, but are not yet in a sexual relationship, touch can be electric. An unexpected contact can bring surprising sexual feelings in response. In the phase before a relationship has become sexual, socially appropriate touch can be a tantalising game that couples play. Working out the type of touch that is acceptable to each woman is part of the task of every lesbian relationship.

Touching is one of the essential lesbian sexual delights. A basic part of touching is holding: holding hands, holding her breasts, cupping her vulva, holding her backside, holding other parts of her body, holding her in your arms. Also lying, sitting, standing together front to front, full length body-to-body, or front to back, like spoons. Being held leads to feelings of comfort and security. It may also lead to unpleasant feelings of constraint if it is not fully consented to. There is a skill in communicating what feels agreeable to you.

Cuddling and snuggling are softer types of holding. These words refer to holding with some kisses, strokes and other caresses thrown in. Stroking refers to long touches that pass over a length over your partner's body. You can stroke her back, her tummy, and her little finger. Strokes can be soft and light, or firm or deep.

Kissing is also basic. Many women find that it is one of the most important elements of lovemaking. You can kiss ears, necks, shoulders, all the way down her spine, sides, crooks of arms, elbows, armpits, collarbones, breasts, nipples, navels, ankles, backs of legs, inner thighs and genitals (see below under oral sex).

Kisses can be feather-light. They can be a little wet with a bit of tongue or they can be very deep and wet. Kisses may be of varying intensity, from soft and gentle through to hot, passionate and insistent.

It is important to be able to breathe while you are kissing. Keep your nose unobstructed. You should make sure that both of you enjoy what is happening. It may sound trite, but not everyone enjoys the same thing. Most women like kisses, but not everyone enjoys deep, wet kisses.

Licking is another thing that you can do with your tongue. You can lick all of the planes, crevices and orifices of her body. Your can pour chocolate sauce, honey or liqueur on her and lick it off. You can lick her ear lobes, the base of her spine and the place between her vulva and her inner thigh.

If you both happen to be at opposite ends of a bath (preferably with incense, music, candles and lots of bubbles, plus or minus champagne), you might like to take her left foot in your hands and gently lick in between each of her toes. She may like to nibble and lick the sole of your foot and ankle.

> **EMMA:** *One of the most erotic things I have ever felt was Julia's tongue sliding in and out between my toes. It drove me mad when she started to lick all the way up my leg and then kept going back to my toes.*

Sucking is related to, but different from, licking. Imagine what it feels like to have someone gently suck your little finger. Special favourites for sucking include the nipples, ear lobes, neck and clitoris. The pressure created can be a true turn-on.

Touching is not confined to the use of your hands and mouth. Touching your partner's vulva and clitoris with your breast and nipple can be extremely pleasurable for you both.

Many women like the feeling of someone cupping their vulva with warm pressure. This may take place through jeans or pants. Stroking over the top of clothes has a different feel to the touch of skin on skin and contains the promise of what is to come. Stroking through thin knickers is another different and highly pleasurable sensation. It may be used to tease, before the eventual delight when the knickers are removed.

Playing gently with the pubic hair and the pubic mound may be a precursor to opening the lips of the vagina and starting to stroke within them.

The clitoris is extremely sensitive. Touching the clitoris is often one of the core pleasures of lesbian sex. It should be approached gently. It is often best to wait until your partner's lubricating fluids have begun to flow, as touching the clitoris while it is dry can be irritating or painful. Many women prefer a gentle touch.

The clitoris may be touched with the fingers, the lips, the tongue, the breast or nipple, or may be cupped with the whole palm. It may be stroked on one side or the other. It may be gently squeezed. Lots of women like gentle, direct pressure with a circular or back and forth motion. The meeting of the inner lips (labia minora) forms a hood over the top of the clitoris. Gently pulling the hood back exposes the glans (see Fig. 3). The end of the glans may be stimulated with tongue or finger. Some women gain most pleasure from stimulation of the glans, or end of the clitoris; others prefer stimulation of the shaft. The sides may be caressed or squeezed. As excitement heightens, a woman who cannot tolerate strong stimulation may find that she wants more intense stroking or touching.

The 'legs' or crura of the clitoris run along the pubic bones and end in the deep spongy tissues. This means that stimulation along both the front and back walls inside the vagina may cause pleasurable sensations in the clitoris. The clitoris may also be stimulated internally via the rectum.

Massage

Massage is a method of treating painful muscles by stroking, kneading, pressing, tapping and other forms of touch. It can also be used just for the physical pleasure it provides. Erotic massage is usually a slow, sensual process of touching where one or more people give pleasure to a single recipient. Many couples gain great delight from sensual massage. The masseuse determines the pace of the process and may use slow titillation to heighten her partner's sensitivity.

When a couple has agreed that one partner will be the passive recipient, a skilful masseuse can repeatedly bring her partner close to orgasm and then let her return to the plateau state. This may cause the eventual orgasmic release to have enormous intensity. In many cultures, erotic massage has been practised as a skilled art. However, gentle touch and good intentions will make a beginner's efforts highly appreciated. A warm room, candlelight and erotic aromatherapy oils such as ylang ylang and musk can add to the effects.

It is very important that the couple agree that the massage will be a sensual massage before the process starts. It can feel invasive to have an ordinary therapeutic massage turn into a sensual massage if this has not been previously agreed to.

Tribadism

This is another form of touching. It involves rubbing genitals together, or rubbing the genitals of one person against the body of another. The word 'tribade' was used by the French and was derived from a Latin word, which meant 'to rub'. It is of particular importance to lesbians because in the nineteenth century lesbians were called 'tribades'. In the erotic novels of the day, this was thought to be the main sexual activity of lesbian women. The thrusting contact of genital areas is also called 'frottage', 'humping' and 'bonking'. Many women enjoy orgasm through this activity and have never heard the names. The full body-to-body contact is exciting. Variations include cunt-to-cunt contact by using a 'scissors' position and taking one of your partner's legs between both of your own. Other variations include rubbing your vulva over any part of your partner's body – the breasts, buttocks and mouth are a few possibilities.

> **JEAN:** *I guess tribadism has always been one of the main ways that I reach orgasm. I find it really extremely erotic. The sensuality is not only in my pelvis and vagina, but in my breasts. Also I feel like I can keep in emotional contact with my partner. It works for me.*

There are two wonderful things about tribadism: it leaves your hands and mouths free to do other things, and you can do it fully clothed.

Oral sex

'Oral sex' means stimulation of the genitals or anus of one partner by the mouth or tongue of the other. The variations of oral sex are limited only by the imagination.

One possible approach is to lick from the inner thighs to the outside of the outer lips gently parting them with your tongue. Explore the inner lips. Lick or suck the clitoris. The clitoris may be tantalised with soft, wet strokes. It may also be tongue-lashed with short, intense strokes or long, vigorous ones. Gently insert your tongue into her vagina. She may enjoy having her perineum licked. It may be okay to use teeth gently but not all women like this. Many women enjoy pressure from a well-placed chin.

There are a number of different positions that women enjoy. Oral sex may occur with one partner sitting or standing and the other kneeling. It can occur in the famous '69' position. She can kneel and straddle your head. In this position, the recipient has the added stimulation of an extremely erotic view of her partner's actions.

Some women have simultaneous oral sex; others find that they are unable to concentrate on both giving and receiving at the same time. Penetration during oral sex may be an added turn-on. Some women love a finger or dildo placed inside the vagina or anus while oral stimulation continues. However, for some women this may be distracting.

Occasionally women at first find the smell or taste of another's vagina unappealing. Others find it very erotic. If you would like to try oral sex, but are not comfortable with the smells or tastes, you and your partner may like to experiment with ways of modifying them. Sex straight after a bubble bath is one option. Lubricating her well with your saliva is a way of putting your own smells and tastes into the situation. Another is to add flavour. Canned spray cream (with or without strawberries), chocolate bars, your favourite liqueur, honey and chocolate sauce are a few options.

One of the difficulties that must be overcome during oral sex is to ensure that the partner who is using her mouth also continues to breathe. In the height of passion it is worthwhile to ensure that your nose is unobstructed. Practice makes perfect. In time this can become second nature.

> **SAM:** *It's an old joke that every lesbian wants to find a partner who can breathe through her ears, but sometimes I think Fiona must be able to. She's so skilful, and sometimes she stays down there driving me crazy for so long.*

> **FIONA:** *It took me a while to learn how, but I've found out that if I just tilt my head at just the right angle I can breathe without any problems. I also learned to pace myself, going from vigorous licking to gentle, soft tongue movements. I found that if I didn't, my tongue and jaw ached. Once I learned how to vary the speed and intensity of what I do I can go on almost forever. I love it.*

If you do get a tired jaw or sore tongue, stop and do something different! Oral sex is not for everyone:

> **JEAN:** *I don't like oral sex. The main reason is because I really like hugs and cuddles. I don't like it when Rosa is down there between my legs. I can't see her face and I can't hold her in my arms. We've tried other positions but they don't work for us, so we rarely do it.*

Some women are very comfortable with oral sex while either they or their partner are menstruating. They consider that a small amount of blood is just another taste. Some enjoy the 'womanliness' of it. Others are repelled by the idea. Inserting a tampon may solve the problem. Or it may be that as a couple, you prefer other sexual activities while one of you is menstruating.

Some women have questions about the hygienic aspects of oral sex. Except when a woman has an infection, the vagina is no 'dirtier' than the average mouth. Both mouths and vaginas contain normal flora (bacteria). These cause no harm and in fact are normal and healthy. If an infection is present, other issues arise (see Chapter 5).

There is another confronting aspect to oral sex. Sometimes women find it difficult to lie back and receive such intimate attention. This may be because we have been repeatedly told as children that our vaginas are dirty and we should not touch them. Also, we have been taught that our role as women is to give pleasure to others. This can make it difficult for us to relax and receive pleasure.

> **JOAN:** *I didn't have any problem with the idea of oral sex, the thought of it really excited me, but every time my partner tried it with me, I kept thinking that I should be doing something too. It was impossible for me to just lie there and accept the pleasure. I would reach down and stroke her shoulders and neck, but this took my mind off what was happening to me. It was only much later, when I realised that I felt guilty about just receiving the pleasure, that I was able to allow myself to accept it. Even now, Dot sometimes has to remind me to 'just enjoy it'.*

> **VI:** *I absolutely adore oral sex. Everyone has a different smell and a different taste. I love giving it and I love being licked. It makes me wet just thinking about it. I particularly love positions where I can see what my lover's tongue is doing. Sitting on a chair, standing, and kneeling with my legs on each side of her face work well for me.*

Ultimately, oral sex is a matter of personal taste. If you don't like it, don't do it. If think you might enjoy it, there are an infinite number of ways to experiment.

Anal sex

Anal sex is any activity that causes pleasure by stimulating the anus. The anus and the area around it are highly erogenous zones. The area between the buttocks, and in fact all of the buttocks can become highly sensitised. Stroking and cupping the buttocks may be a nice prelude to more intimate activity.

The anus may be licked. Gently licking or sucking all the way around it is called 'rimming'. It may be touched or stroked. If it has not already been licked then a little lubricant (your own readily available saliva, or any other water-soluble lubricant) may make the sensations more highly erotic. If your partner feels happy about it, gently inserting a finger in and out of the anus may be pleasurable. The nerve endings are mostly around the entrance, so most women feel that there's not much to be gained by deep penetration. Others, however, are really turned on by the feeling of fullness. Some enjoy the penetration of their anus by toys or dildos.

Like the vagina, the anus may expand when you are excited. Under conditions of high arousal, it may readily accept more than one finger, and even a whole fist (see 'Fisting').

The anal sphincter is a strong muscle, and since it ensures that faeces stays where it ought to, it is important not to damage it. Anal sex should therefore always start slowly and gently to ensure that the recipient is aroused, and the anal sphincter is relaxed and open to penetration.

You may be put off by a worry about faeces, germs or smells. Some women incorporate baths, showers and enemas as part of their foreplay. A warm stream of water can be very exciting. Others simply choose not to worry.

> **SAM:** *I really like anal sex, but I thought it was dirty. Also, I was worried that it could damage me. Then one day, a friend of mine (who is a doctor) happened to mention that they actually put people to sleep and stretch their anuses to fix some anal and rectal health problems. She said anal sex can actually be good for you! After that I just stopped worrying and enjoyed it.*

If you do engage in anal sex, it is important that you do not touch your partner's vagina with a hand or finger that has been touching her anus. If you do, you may put her at risk of urinary tract or vaginal infections by transferring bacteria from one location to another. It is important to realise that it is possible to pass infections between partners by anal sex. It is possible to transmit Hepatitis A and B (and also Hepatitis C and HIV if there is bleeding from any cuts, scratches or injury). See Chapter 5.

Fingering, finger-fucking, fisting

Fingering and finger-fucking refer to putting a finger or fingers inside your partner's vagina or anus. In the past, some lesbians have judged these activities as being 'too heterosexual' or 'copying what men do.' Some women do not like having anything put inside them. They may have suffered previous sexual abuse, or they may simply prefer not to have their intimate space invaded. Women may feel differently about sexual penetration at different times in their menstrual cycle. Not only do emotional responses vary, but also the cervix may drop lower during menstruation, making penetration less comfortable.

Many women adore the feeling of their partner's fingers inside them, filling their vagina. Others love the feeling of a finger moving in and out of their anus. Fingering can cause pleasure through stimulation of the vagina and cervix or through the movements it causes in the clitoris. It can also be used to stimulate the G spot (see Appendix 2 for how to do this).

> **JOAN:** *I've had several lovers who could ejaculate when I fingered them, especially when I fingered their G spots. It's never happened to me. I love the feeling that I can bring a woman to such pleasure that she ejaculates. You get this flood of liquid on your fingers and hand.*

'Fisting' refers to the insertion of the whole fist into the vagina or anus. If a woman is highly aroused, and particularly if she has had children, her vagina may accommodate a fist. However, if you are post-menopausal, or for any other reason have fragile vaginal tissues, this activity is probably not for you. Women who want to receive their partner's fist may find that what was initially impossible becomes easy in a state of high arousal. It may be part of gentle lovemaking. It may also play a part in BDSM (Bondage, Domination, Sadism & Masochism) or more intense consensual sex. Some women enjoy 'giving or getting it rough'.[7] This does not mean thrusting inconsiderately. Reckless behaviour can cause damage and pain. Fisting needs to be done by a careful lover so it is often suggested that both partners be drug- and alcohol-free. These substances tend to cause decreased awareness of pain, and reduce a person's capacity to act with care for their partner's well-being.

If you want to try vaginal fisting, make sure your partner is well aroused, and agrees that she wants to do it. Do not wear any jewellery! Use gloves for safe sex. Start with either oral sex, or fingering her, or both. Ensure that there is lots of lube, both on your hand and on her vulva and vagina. Start with one or two fingers inside her, moving with her movements. As she relaxes and opens, increase the number of fingers inside her to three or four. Continue moving with her. She may be exerting a fair amount of pressure on your hand. When you are going to move so that your whole fist is inside her, your palm should be facing upwards, press inside, tucking your thumb in, and making your hand into a fist in one smooth movement. You shouldn't need any force! Either she is able to easily accommodate your fist or she isn't. If you use force you may cause her harm! The hand can be moved in a twisting or screwing motion, or in and out, as gently or forcefully as your partner desires.

Some women like to have the hand removed gently after orgasm, other like it to be removed quickly at the point of orgasm to give a different sensation. The feeling of having someone's fist inside you can be emotionally overwhelming. The orgasms can be extremely intense. The feeling of intimacy that permits a whole hand to be inside your lover can also be emotionally breathtaking. Couples often need quiet time together to come down from the profound emotional high.

Some women say that the secret to fisting is communication.

LISA: *We don't do fisting often, it's like a new frontier for us. You have to really trust someone to let her put a whole hand in you. There's no way I'd consider doing it with a man. To*

*make it work we have to talk a lot, like, 'I've got three
finger's in you now, does it feel okay?' 'Do you want another
finger in there now?' 'Are you ready for all of my hand?' If
we didn't talk like that, there's no way we could do it. To let
someone put their fist in you, you have to be absolutely open
and vulnerable. An orgasm when you are so open, and so
filled up, is mind-blowing. It's made me feel like I was about
to pass out. The feeling of being allowed to have your whole
hand in someone is also phenomenal. Having your lover's
vagina spasming on your fist when she orgasms just blows
me away. It's the most absolutely emotionally intense high I
can imagine.*

For anal fisting, unless you are happy to play in faeces (this is known
as 'scat'), enemas may be part of foreplay. Again, the receiver must be
absolutely relaxed. Anal fisting can cause permanent damage to the
anal sphincter, so both women must take great care.

Both vaginal and anal fisting are more likely to cause bleeding than
most other types of lesbian sexual activity. If you intend to try either of
these, it is a good idea to be familiar with the safe sex practices set out
in Chapter 5.

Sex toys

Sex toys have been used by lesbian and heterosexual women since the
beginning of human history.

Dildos are made to insert into the vagina or anus. They come in an
astounding array of colours, sizes and shapes. They are available in
plastic, silicone and a large number of other substances, including steel.
The lesbian community has, at times, had an uneasy relationship with
them.

ANNE: *Some lesbians are not interested in dildos and
vibrators. You know, they say things like 'If you want a penis,
why aren't you with a man, why do you want to use a fake*

one?' When Lucy and I got our first dildo we felt guilty about it. It was a secret. It was a large double-ended one and it didn't work very well. It was too big for us. We'd try and use it and it would fall out. We'd either end up getting frustrated or just fall in a heap laughing. It ended up in the bottom of the wardrobe. Now we go to shops with sex gear designed by women for women. We like experimenting. In the last few years, we have bought a vibrator and another dildo with a harness. They've been much more successful. I might use the vibrator anywhere on her body – nipples, backside, clitoris, cunt. The dildo is a much smaller, soft, silicone one. We only use it occasionally, but it's nice because with the harness it leaves your hands free. We use it with lots of lube. Because it's silicone, it warms up as it slides in and out. Very erotic. I have to say, it gives me a different feeling having sex with it. We both like it.

ANDREA: I've always seen myself as butch. When I came out forty years ago, I mixed with a group of women who taught me how butches were supposed to behave. We were the tough ones. We didn't talk much about 'packing'. That was wearing a dildo with a harness ready to use. I wouldn't let a partner touch me sexually. I would rarely take my clothes off at all during sex. I would just do it to her. I've lived through the whole feminist scene where that was a problem. These days it's fine to talk about this stuff. Now I think it's more important to just enjoy who I am.

Many women delight in the different sensations that sex toys can provide.

LE-ANNE: I absolutely love the things you can buy. I think the best thing I ever did was get a vibrator. It makes me independent. One of the most sensual things we do is use it together. We use a condom on it and change it. Nina will use

> *it on the outside of my cunt lips, then between them with lots*
> *of lube, then inside me. It really gets me going.*

Some dildos are curved to stimulate the G-Spot. Some are double-ended to be used by partners. They come with ribbed and textured surfaces. Dildos may be purchased with a variety of harnesses. Vibrators also come in many varieties, including double-ended ones for couples.

Dildos that have been designed for use in the anus are called 'butt plugs'. These have a different shape to vaginal dildos, often having a flared or flat end that is designed to prevent the toy being inserted too far up the rectum and getting stuck. There are good reasons for using a specially designed toy for anal play. The rectum is connected to the large intestine and there are many medical stories about objects that have been inserted too far into the colon. It is not unknown for people to require an operating theatre procedure to remove foreign objects. Using a special toy for the anus also helps prevent transmission of germs from the rectum to the vagina and therefore minimises the risk of infection.

Other toys specifically designed for the anus include 'strings of beads'. These are modern copies of an ancient Asian erotic implement. There may be up to six beads on a durable, washable cord. They vary in size from strings with six pea-sized balls, to balls of golf ball dimensions and larger. The 'beads' are inserted into the anus during sexual activity. Traditionally, they are pulled out either slowly or quickly at the moment of orgasm. They are said to greatly intensify the feelings.

Vibrators may be an adjunct to masturbation, or may add different sensations to a couple's sex play. They may be especially designed for either the vagina or anus. 'Lube', or lubricant, is an essential adjunct to the use of many sex toys. It comes in a large number of types and flavours.

> **ANNE:** *I love lube, it's taken the pressure out of sex for me.*
> *Before I discovered it I used to worry that I wasn't getting wet*
> *enough. I felt that my partner would think I wasn't hot for*
> *her. I would be really turned on, but I wouldn't have any*

vaginal juices. I used to stress out about it. Now I just make
sure that there's a heap of lube down there. No one can tell
that I might be dry. Feels like freedom.

There are many reasons why normal women may not have enough
vaginal juices to make sex comfortable. Lube solves the problem. It
makes the use of sex toys easy. It is essential in safe sex (see Chapter 5).
Lube also has erotic dimensions all of its own.

> **SANDRA:** *Sometimes Ros will put lots of lube all over my
> cunt and arsehole. She uses one finger in and out of my cunt,
> and one finger in and out of my arse. I love the feeling of her
> fingers, but more than anything I love the slippery squishy
> feeling of the lube.*

Nipple clips and clamps are created to apply controlled pressure. Some
see them as tools for those who are interested in BDSM (see below),
however, many lesbians enjoy the sensations that they provide.

There are a large variety of other toys available. These are often
copies of very ancient courtesans' devices. Ben-wa balls are inserted
and worn in the vagina. The weight and movement of these balls
provides stimulation. More modern technology has produced battery-
powered vibrating balls that may be worn all day. Leather and erotic
lingerie are also part of lesbian sensuality.

You do not have to frequent a commercial sex shop in order to find
sex toys. Chocolate bars, chocolate biscuits, chocolate eclairs, candles,
fruit (bananas) vegetables (zucchinis, cucumbers, carrots), hairbrush
handles, deodorant bottles, golf balls, craft beads and gearshifts from
cars are just a few of the home-made improvised dildos that I have been
told about. If you are being creative with a homemade substitute, take
care with your choice of object. Don't use anything with sharp edges, or
anything brittle that could break inside you with over enthusiastic use.

Feathers are an eternal favourite for sexual pleasure. You can buy
expensive ones in sex shops, or you can pull them out of the feather
duster your mum has had for years. A silk scarf can substitute for the
specially made satin or leather blindfolds, which add to anticipation, as

the person wearing the blindfold does not know what the next sensation will be. Nylon stockings can substitute for commercially available handcuffs if an urge to investigate restraint is unexpectedly upon you (make sure you don't tie them too tightly). Chocolate ice-cream topping is a great substitute for expensive chocolate body-paint.

BDSM

BD is short for bondage and discipline or domination. Sub/dom is short for submission and domination and is about exploring power relationships. It may or may not contain sexual activity. SM comes from the sadomasochism and refers to sexual activity that intensifies sexual pleasure through pain.

A recurrent discussion among the community that enjoys these practices is 'what to call ourselves'. SM and BDSM are currently used abbreviations.

Particularly in our larger cities, many Australian lesbians are investigating SM, sub/dom and BD. Some see SM and sub/dom as intrinsically linked. Others see them as separate and feel that mixing the terms up is not helpful to understanding the type of activities that are enjoyed.

Both sub/dom and SM may use bondage or restraint. They utilise some of the same toys: blindfolds, hoods, gags, handcuffs and chains. Some toys are specially designed to create pain. These include nipple clips, clit clips, paddles and whips. Hot candle wax is used to create pain without scarring. Some SM lesbians enjoy 'blood sports'. This may involve piercing or scarifying (cutting designs in the skin surface to produce permanent or semi-permanent scars).

Lesbians who are into SM are often vigilant about safe sex. Negotiation of the type of activities which will occur, and consent, are seen as vitally important. The person receiving the pain has a safe word or visual signal that is used to stop the activity.

SM and sub/dom elicit a variety of responses from lesbians. There has been much discussion and debate about them. Women involved in the SM scene assert that the activity of consenting adults should not be a cause for comment. Other women feel extremely challenged or threatened by the activities. Some argue that there are political implications for the whole culture.

SUSAN: *I found it really disturbing when SM stuff started appearing at Mardi Gras. When I lived in Sydney, I was in a meeting of gay people that was invaded by neo-nazis and I had to run for my life (literally).*

I was upset when things that looked violent started appearing in our community. As a feminist I felt that I'd worked all my life against the presence of power difference in my sexual relationships. I reacted against SM strongly. Over the years I've listened to what SM lesbians say about how they feel marginalised in our community. I've come to a place where I'm tired of all types of intolerance and I just want to live and let live. What they do doesn't bother me any more.

ZOE: *I got into SM because I was curious. Also, I love all sorts of sensations at the same time. I'm into sensuality. The idea of pleasure through pain didn't seem strange to me. Anyone who goes jogging or does any kind of endurance sport can tell you about what it's like when the endorphins kick in. And when you think about it, it's not that unusual in our culture. Many of our great accomplishments (like reaching the North Pole, for example), were achieved by women or men who were prepared to suffer.*

JULIE: *No way, I'd hate it. I got bashed enough as a child. I could never find any pleasure in it.*

ELLEN: *We're playing round the edges of it I guess. We're experimenting with tying each other up, blindfolds and 'soft' pain, like an ice block dildo on the clitoris or used anally. Even the feelings that come up with that level of helplessness are pretty challenging.*

SANDRA: *No-one who is not involved has the right to comment. You have no idea what is involved. There is an enormous amount of responsibility and often preparation. When I am a bottom and give over my power, it takes ultimate trust. When I am a top I am creative. I am also responsible, nurturing and knowledgeable. It takes a huge amount of energy to be responsible for yourself, and also for another person's body and mind. It takes endurance and maturity.*

If you are interested in knowing more about BDSM please see the Resources section for a list of books and websites. Some women may feel a little shy at the idea of ordering these books from their local retailer. However, The Darlinghurst Bookshop, Sydney (listed in Resources) will be able to supply you with many books on this topic. This bookshops stocks new releases as they become available.

Other erotica

It is obvious that the ways women can enjoy sensual and sexual activity together are limited only by imagination. Having been privileged in being able to talk to lots of lesbians, it seems to me that we have an aptitude for creativity. Lesbians enjoy phone sex, exhibitionism, voyeurism, erotic literature and videos. Some like group sex. We enjoy the sensuality of water. We love sex in baths and spas. We enjoy the additional pleasure that is provided by the locations where we are sexual. We make love under the moon and in the open air. Some enjoy the feeling of pounding and helplessness that comes from making love in the surf and in the place at the water's edge on beaches. We use the pressure of jets of water from taps and hoses. We enjoy simply showering together on weekday mornings.

Some enjoy the titillation of strip tease. Many like a variety of sexual positions. A few enjoy 'scat'; others enjoy 'water sports' or 'golden showers' (sexual activity with urine). Some women use drugs (amyl nitrate, ecstasy, alcohol, marijuana and others) during sexual activity.

Many women find a spiritual connection through sexuality. Some investigate erotic spirituality techniques and traditions to learn how to heighten sensitivity. For large numbers of lesbian women, however, sexual activity is an enjoyable domestic event that does not contain anything exotic.

In all the sexual activities that we explore, it is important for each woman to find her 'comfort zone'. Sexual interaction can provide comfort, joy and intense pleasure. In order to know what you like, you have to know yourself. You need to be able to honour yourself. You must believe that you deserve pleasure and can get what you want. As women explore the sexual parts of their personalities, they also find out more about who they are. The capacity to ask for what you want, and to be pleasured or nurtured, spills over into everyday life. The joy of deep connection with another flows into the way you live in the world.

5

Sexual Health

Health workers often see 'Sexual Health' as referring to healthy sexual organs. Although physical health is very important, I believe sexual health also includes emotional, intellectual and spiritual components.

Emotional sexual health involves feeling good about yourself. This enables you to value the gift that you are giving when you have sex with someone. You may be choosing to have sex because you want fun, exercise and an orgasm. Or you may be choosing to have sex because you want to give and receive the privilege of intimate contact. Either way, what you are giving is valuable. Women who are healthy emotionally value themselves. Women who feel worthless or hopeless find it difficult to have respect for themselves. It therefore becomes difficult to ensure that others treat them with respect.

A healthy emotional base for sex involves being able to work out what you do want and being able to ask for it. It involves being able to identify what you don't want, and saying 'no' to it. Emotional health permits compromise that feels comfortable to you and allows you to prevent yourself from being pushed into things you don't want to do. A woman who is emotionally healthy sets limits about what is and is not alright with her. She knows her boundaries.

Intellectual sexual health is about having a knowledge base. There is a lot to know about sex. You can choose to learn a little or a lot. It can be helpful to know how your body works. It is also a very good idea to be aware of the risks that are involved in sex. This book and the resources section provide a very good starting place to gather information.

Spiritual sexual health is something that not all women care about. Many women feel that it is irrelevant to their lives. A clear decision that sex has no spiritual significance may be as healthy for some as a choice to honour and investigate this aspect of sexuality.

Sexual health may involve an acknowledgment that sex has a spiritual dimension. It may also mean ensuring that the actions you take are congruent with the deeper significance that sexuality has for you. The meaning that sex has spiritually will vary for each woman. Some women see it as part of their life's task to investigate this. The resources section lists books about sex and spirituality.

PHYSICAL SEXUAL HEALTH

Sexual health check-ups and Pap tests

A sexual health check-up for women offers a physical examination, and tests to identify sexually transmitted infections. The tests include blood tests, vaginal swabs, cervical swabs and sometimes urine tests. The check-up also gives you a chance to talk to a health worker about sexual issues. Pap tests are part of a woman's sexual health check-up. All women should have a Pap test every two years. In the past, many lesbians believed that they didn't need to have Pap tests. Doctors believed the same thing.

JOAN: *I'm almost 50 so I went to my doctor to have a Pap test. It took every bit of courage I had to front up. When I told her what I had come for, she said, 'Joan, I didn't think*

> *you'd been sexually active'. She has known me for a long*
> *time, and she knew that there was no man in my life. It took*
> *everything I had to say 'I've been in a relationship with Dot*
> *for years'. She sort of flinched and sat back in her chair, got*
> *a very embarrassed look on her face and said, 'If you haven't*
> *had intercourse with a man, you don't need one'. She*
> *wouldn't do a Pap test for me. I went out of there feeling like*
> *I was a leper. I haven't been able to go back.*

The belief that lesbians don't need Pap tests is wrong! Human papilloma virus, which is one of the causes of cervical cancer, is common in lesbian women. Smoking is another risk factor for cervical cancer. Many lesbians have either had sex with men in the past or still have sex with men. Women who are HIV positive should have Pap tests every six months.

The purpose of the Pap test is to detect early changes in the cells on the cervix that occur before cancer of the cervix develops. Regular Pap tests reduce a woman's risk of developing cancer of the cervix by 90 per cent.

> **CATH:** *When I go for a Pap test, I also ask for an STI screen,*
> *just so I know where I stand. I have always had a check-up*
> *after relationships have ended. I've also had check-ups when*
> *I've been considering getting into a new relationship.*

STI (sexually transmitted infection) check-ups are a good idea if you have had unsafe sex. Some women like to have check-ups so that they can say to a new lover: 'I've had a check-up – have you had one?'

However, if you go for a Pap test, the doctor or health care worker will not always do the full sexually transmitted infection screen. Believe it or not, doctors are sometimes embarrassed to ask women about their sexual activity. So if a woman asks for a Pap test, sometimes that is exactly what the doctor may do. Doctors will not always say 'Are you at risk for other sexually transmitted infections, should I do a sexually transmitted infection screen?' In fact, if a doctor does do STI tests without discussing it with you, that may constitute an assault. If you want an STI screen and the doctor doesn't mention the issue, it is important for you to raise the subject.

Unless you go to a woman's health centre, sexual health clinic or a Family Planning Association clinic for your Pap test, you may have to say 'I want a sexually transmitted infection screen too'.

Finding a health practitioner

Lesbians often say that they have difficulty choosing a doctor. Recent research suggests that lesbians want health workers to ask questions in ways that affirm that same-sex relationships are normal, for instance, 'Do you have a partner?' rather than 'Do you have a boyfriend?'. We take our cues from the way the health worker or doctor behaves. If what the practitioner says indicates that she/he doesn't really notice that homosexual people exist in the world, we will be more likely not to give any details about our sexual preference or home life. If the health worker gives some indication that same-sex sexual activity is one of the ranges of normal choices, we are much more likely to feel comfortable about discussing our concerns with her/him.

> **CARA:** *I had persistent stomach pain and got my GP, who knew I was a dyke, to refer me to a gastroenterologist. He took my medical history and then asked if I had a partner. I said yes. He asked some other question that assumed my partner was a man. I took a deep breath and said 'She's...'. That was it. I could not get him off the subject of my relationship. He was asking all sorts of questions that had nothing to do with my health. I felt he was improper and intrusive. Even if he hadn't been so over the top with it all, I didn't feel like it was my job to educate him about my lifestyle. I expected that doctors would be taught at least a bit about us. I was really angry about that. He didn't organise any appropriate tests for me. He just prescribed some medication and said to come back in three months. My GP was disgusted that he hadn't organised the things she had*

asked him to do. She was shocked when I told her about the conversation.

SAM: *When I go to a doctor I want to feel safe. I want to be able to talk about my life without feeling like a freak or without being judged.*

Women's health centres often have lesbian-friendly doctors. Ask your friends about doctors who have been helpful. Also, check p. 245 in the resources chapter.

Safe sex

'Safe sex' is the way to prevent the spread of STIs. Until recently lesbian women have not had much information about the transmission of infections through lesbian sexual practices. Many of us started thinking and talking about these issues as a result of HIV. However, the practical reality is that other sexually transmitted organisms are far more prevalent. Herpes, vaginosis, genital warts and hepatitis are much more of a real risk for women who have sex with women.

> **JOANNE:** *I never worried about 'precautions'. We used to say that the only people less likely to get a sexual infection than lesbians were nuns. I've had to rethink it since my friend got Hep B. I'm really glad that at the moment I'm in a stable relationship. Both of us have had tests, and are clear.*

In the past, lesbians (and their doctors) believed that the risk of sexually transmitted infections was much higher for heterosexual women. A recent Australian study indicates that this is not true. Dr Katherine Fethers and others analysed data from medical records of 2831 women who attended the Sydney Sexual Health Clinic between 1991 and 1998.[1] Women who have sex with women (WSW)[2] are just as at risk of STIs as heterosexual women. They are at increased risk of bacterial vaginosis. For detailed information about the various STIs, see Appendix 3.

Women who have sex with women may also have sex with men, or have done so in the past. One of the ways that infections spread is through intravenous drug use (IDU). Some lesbian women use injectable drugs. An infection acquired by IDU can be passed on by sex.

Do I want to be safe?

This is a personal decision for every woman. Health workers and sex educators no longer assume that we will all choose to be safe.

Decisions about safe sex are in some ways similar to decisions about swimming. Lots of people never swim in anything deeper than a bathtub. Many people swim in the surf. Others choose to go deep sea diving. Some deliberately choose to dive where they know they will see sharks. A small number pay to dive where they can feed sharks. It's all about lifestyle choices. There are degrees of risk. Occasionally someone drowns in the surf. Every so often a shark bites a scuba diver. Rarely, a shark kills someone. Lots of surfers and many scuba divers will tell you that the risk is worth it for the joy of the experience. However, the majority of people choose not to put their lives in jeopardy.

The important thing is to be informed about the seriousness of the risks, and to make your decisions consciously, not in the heat of the moment.

If you sit quietly and ask yourself 'How much risk do I like to have in my life?', an answer will probably spring to mind. It is important to know your boundaries and your limits. It is also important to ensure that both you and other people respect them.

Sex educators argue that the risks of unprotected casual sex are substantial. They maintain that safe sex can be so enjoyable, and will decrease the risks so much, that it is worth it.

How safe?

Advisers from different countries express varying views in their recommendations about safe sex. In the United States, health educators talk about risk *elimination*. They advise women to use barriers on all occasions of sexual contact, except in long-term monogamous relationships where both partners have had clear sexually transmitted infection (STI) tests. In England, health workers from the Bernhard Clinic for Lesbian Health speak about risk reduction. They suggest that women weigh up their particular activities and decide what degree of risk they are willing to take.

I have listened to women talk about their attitudes to safe sex. It seems to me that many women who intend a long-term relationship with one person prefer to make an assessment of the particular risks, and then to make a decision about safe sex practices. Women who like to have sex with lots of different partners are often very well educated about safe sex methods and use them routinely.

SEXUALLY TRANSMITTED INFECTIONS

The problem

STIs can be split into two categories: the serious life-threatening ones (hepatitis viruses and HIV), and those that are not life-threatening.

Any activity which lets body fluids from one person get into the body of another has a chance of passing on a serious sexually transmitted infection. Blood-to-blood contact (for example, menstrual blood into an open cut, or sharing needles to inject drugs), and male ejaculate to a broken mucus membrane, carry the highest risk of transmitting life-threatening infections. Mucus membranes are the tender, porous surfaces that are found inside the mouth, vagina, anus and nose, and on the moist surfaces of the eyes.

Lesbians are believed to have an extremely low risk of HIV transmission. At the time of writing, there have been only a handful of cases recorded in world medical literature where the method of transmission appears to be woman-to-woman sexual practice. Hepatitis is, however, not uncommon (see p.222 in Appendix 3).

Lesbians much more frequently contract warts, herpes and 'BV' (bacterial vaginosis) from each other. We may also transmit candida, chlamydia, which can cause infertility, and other organisms by our sexual activities. (The individual infections that can be contracted are discussed in Appendix 2.) Safe sex practices reduce the risk. These infections are considered by some to be 'less serious' because they are not life-threatening. Some women have these infections and are not troubled by them. Others find that the infection makes their life miserable.

Some of the 'less serious' organisms are capable of being transmitted by touch. Touching your partner's vagina or vulva after touching your own can pass infections. Rubbing your vulva against your partner's vulva can also transmit them. Fingers, sex toys and other objects can transmit organisms.

Prevention

If you want to ensure that you won't catch a serious sexually transmitted infection, you will have to prevent the body fluids of any other person getting into your body. This is the same for both lesbians and heterosexual women. However, herpes and warts can be transmitted just from skin on skin contact. It is not known how to prevent this, except by choosing not to have contact.

The only other way to be safe is to check that neither partner has an infection. This is an option if you only have sex with one person. It will only protect you from infection if you both agree not to have sex with other people (as contact with others can expose both of you to risk). If you choose this option, you may both have a set of sexually transmitted infection tests. The HIV test will need to be repeated three months later. This test should be repeated because the AIDS virus can be present in the blood stream in such low quantities that it does not show up on the first test. This is called 'the window period'. Having a second test after the window period has passed means that if the virus is present, it will probably be detected. In addition, some organisms (like chlamydia) can be difficult to find. Repeating certain tests gives peace of mind that you have the 'all clear'.

The only way to be absolutely sure that you won't get a sexually transmitted disease is to be celibate, or to be in a monogamous relationship with a woman who has had clear STI tests. You would need to be certain that your partner had not had sex with anyone else. Even in this situation, one of you can get thrush, or recurrence of genital herpes that you contracted years ago and didn't know that you had. These can be passed on, so even in monogamous relationships, it can be necessary to think about safe sex practice.

Safe/unsafe sexual activities

Safe

Closed mouth kissing (unless one of you has a cold sore), hugging, massage, masturbation, including watching each other masturbate or masturbating together (each woman touching only herself), rubbing bodies against each other (tribadism) with clothes on, sharing fantasy and talking erotically are all considered to be safe sexual activities.

Probably safe

Deep throat kissing, protected vaginal/oral and anal/oral sex (with lots of lube and a dental dam or other barrier), touching (including penetration using a finger/fist etc in vagina or anus) while wearing a latex glove and using lube, touching without gloves if you are sure you have intact skin, vibrators and dildos that are protected by a condom, are all considered to be unlikely to transmit serious infections.

> **JO:** *I used to think that I would never bother with safe sex. Now, so many of my friends assume that if you have sex casually, it will be safe sex. I've got used to it. In fact, it's really a bit of a turn on. If I'm going out and I've got my lube and latex in my pocket I already feel a bit turned on because I know I'm hunting for a fuck. Once I start to put the gloves on my cunt juices up, because I know what's about to happen.*

Tribadism while unclothed could transmit scabies or lice. These infections are a nuisance, but do not cause long-term harm and are easily treated. There is a chance that unclothed tribadism could transmit genital herpes or warts.

Less safe

Unprotected oral sex may pass on herpes or hepatitis B but is very unlikely to transmit HIV or hepatitis C (unless your partner is menstruating).

The risk of oral sex is that the viruses that transmit the serious diseases (HIV and the hepatitis viruses), may gain entry to your body through broken skin in your mouth. Many women have tiny abrasions on the gums, and around their teeth, or gum disease, that could permit viral entry.

Touching a vagina, vulva or anus without a barrier (unless you are absolutely sure you have clean, intact skin), and using sex toys with no barrier, are all thought to be capable of transmitting infections.

The risk of any of these activities is greater if you or your partner has cuts on your fingers or hands, or broken skin around the anus or genitals. To cause infection, viruses need a way of entering your blood stream. If organisms are present, and you have cuts, or broken skin, the risk of infection is increased. Jagged fingernails increase chance by allowing the possibility of a scratch; short, neatly manicured fingernails reduce risk.

Risk assessment

There is only really one way to gauge the risk of a sexual encounter, and that is to have information. You need to know whether the person you would like to have sex with believes she has a sexually transmissible infection. It helps to know how long it has been since she last had STI tests. It is possible she could have infections that she isn't aware of. Therefore, you also need to know if she has had multiple previous partners, and whether or not some of them have been men, and if she uses (or has used) intravenous drugs. The best way to find out is to talk to your partner. Unfortunately, we all need to remember that people do not always tell the truth.

A person who believes she has no infections, has been monogamous, with few previous partners, has not had sex with men, and who has never used intravenous drugs represents a very low risk.

But not no risk! Even low risk women may have infections they are unaware of.

If you do not know your partner's background and you do not want to risk infection, safe sex still allows sexual pleasure.

How do you do safe sex?

Essentially, safe sex means having a barrier between you and your partner's body fluids. For heterosexuals (and lesbians having sex with men), it's relatively easy; a condom over an erect penis is usually effective. Lesbians who want to have safe sex use 'dams'.

When health workers first began to think that lesbian women might need protection from HIV infection, they recommended that they use 'dental dams'. These are pieces of latex developed by dentists for use in keeping fluids away from the areas that they were working on. If women couldn't get hold of dental dams, it was suggested that they cut up condoms, open them and lie them flat, or cut the palm section from a latex glove. Sex with these barriers was difficult. They got a reputation as being unpleasant and impractical.

Janey and Clive Woodward from the Australian company Kiaora were, at the time, importers of dental dams. They enthusiastically embraced the challenge of developing an appropriate product for sexual use. 'Glyde Dams' were the result. They come in three varieties: wild berry flavoured (which is purple in colour), plain (vanilla), and black (cola). They are super thin, sheer, soft and silky, and are large enough to be useful (24 cm x 15 cm). They allow delicious sensitivity. The Resources section at the back of the book lists retail and other suppliers. They are often freely available at dance parties.

Commercially made leather harnesses to hold them in place are available but they are expensive. I've known enterprising women to cut the crutch out of a pair of knickers and sew a dam in place. Others have adapted stocking suspender belts for the purpose. However, with lube, Glyde dams will often stay where you put them. There is a sort of surface tension effect and they stick!

To use the dam, take it out of its package! (I was told of a couple who didn't realise they had to remove the wrapping.) Moisten one side with water-based lubricant, place the wet side of the dam over the entire vulva or anus, and go for it.

Have plenty of dams on hand. If you switch from vaginal to anal sex, change dams. If you forget which side was in contact with the vulva or anus, change dams. On a rare occasion when vaginal secretions overflow the dam (this doesn't happen so much now that the dams are a more user-friendly size), stop, wipe with tissues, and start again with a new dam.

For finger or fist in vagina, or anal sex, some women choose to use latex gloves. If you have no cuts or breaks in your skin you cannot contract an infection from sexual juices. However, you can pass on an infection if you have touched your own vagina or anus, or your partner's anus, before touching her vagina. Some women have dry skin that is prone to cracking, or have cuts on their hands. Others simply choose not to take any risk. Gloves are widely available at chemists and in supermarkets. Use the thin ones sold in multi packs. Don't go from anal to vaginal sex without changing gloves. If you transfer bacteria from the rectum to the vagina you can cause vaginal and urinary tract infections. For fisting or anal penetration, remember, the key is lots and lots of lube.

Women sometimes wear two gloves on the same hand. This has a number of benefits. You can stimulate your partner's anus, then take the top glove off and move right on to exciting her vagina or clitoris. Also, if in the heat of the moment you happen forget where you were touching her last, you can just whip the top glove off and keep going.

One way to dispose of dams and gloves is to take the used items in a hand that still has a glove on. With the other hand, peel the glove off so it turns inside out and contains the other used items on the inside. Knot the glove, or put it in a knotted plastic bag, and throw it in a bin.

Many women choose not to share sex toys. It's certainly safer if each woman keeps to her own toy. However, if you do plan to share your dildos and vibrators, condoms are a good way of preventing infections being passed from woman to woman. If you think you might use a sex toy for both of you, it's a good idea to start with two condoms on it and take one off when you change the person it's pleasuring. Likewise, if you plan to move from anus to vagina with dildo or vibrator, two condoms are a good idea.

A few don'ts
- Don't forget to check the 'use-by' date on dams and condoms.
- Don't share or re-use dams.
- Don't use latex products if you or your partner is allergic to latex. Non-latex gloves are available at pharmacies. Non-latex dams are being developed.

Special considerations for anal sex
Unlike the vagina, the anus has no capacity to lubricate itself. Also the tissue inside the anus and rectum is tender and not built to withstand friction. It is easy to create small tears and cracks if anal sex is not performed with care and consideration. Use lots and lots of lube and be careful to ensure that you listen to your lover's cues about whether she is enjoying what is happening.

Can cling wrap be used?
Most health educators say that cling wrap or gladwrap is not an effective barrier because it contains 'micro-pores', or little holes, which may let infection through. The Bernhard Clinic for Lesbian Health at Charing Cross Hospital in London advises in its video 'Well Sexy Woman' that the microwaveable type of cling film is an adequate barrier. Australian health educators do not endorse this view. They advise that dams are purpose-made to prevent infection, and we are best to use them!

How do we clean our sex toys?
Wash non-electrical sex toys with water and soap or detergent, and rinse. Then, to disinfect toys (preventing virus transmission), immerse them in a solution that is one part bleach and two parts water for ten minutes. Afterwards, rinse the toy in fresh water and dry it.

Don't immerse vibrators; it may damage or destroy them. Vibrators often have latex or silicon sheaths (and sometimes, detachable balls) that can be slipped off and treated like other sex toys. Use a condom on the vibrator. After use, wipe it over with a wet sponge and detergent, then wipe in a solution that is one part bleach and two parts water, or alternatively a disinfectant solution that is 70 per cent alcohol, then rinse and dry the toy.

Other safety issues

Drugs and alcohol

If you choose to drink alcohol or use drugs, take a moment to think about why you do it. Often people like the way they feel after taking them. It's important to remember that drugs and alcohol are called 'mind-altering substances' for good reason. They affect the way you think and feel. In relation to sex, they affect your judgment.

Women often say they've had sex with someone who they would never have chosen if they were sober or straight. Drugs and alcohol often have an impact on whether people use safe sex. Personally, I don't believe there is any right or wrong about using drugs or alcohol. However, there are consequences. If you think that you might choose to use drugs or alcohol, and you have decided that you prefer safe sex then it is a good idea to prepare ahead of time. Make sure you have dams and lube with you.

Safety issues in relation to drugs and alcohol also include thinking ahead about who you are going to be with when using or drinking, and how you are going to get home safely.

Penetration

Every so often a woman turns up in a hospital emergency department with a foreign object stuck inside her anus or vagina. Occasionally, people turn up with vaginal or anal damage because consensual rough sex got out of hand. It is worth being aware that these things can happen. Give thought to prevention.

If you have a look back at Fig. 5 on p.24, you will notice that the vagina is a dead end. It really is impossible for things to get lost in there. If an object slips inside it is usually possible to insert one or two fingers and get it out. The woman with the object inside her can often get it out simply by 'bearing down', using the muscles in her pelvic floor in a similar way as if she was trying to push a baby out. This is similar to the sort of muscle movement you make to push out faeces when you are straining on the toilet. In fact, sitting on the toilet and pushing is a good way to get a foreign body out of either the rectum or vagina.

The rectum is very different from the vagina. It is not a dead end and things can slip right inside, and can go a long way up the large intestine. You will notice that purpose-made 'butt-plugs' all have a flared end to prevent them slipping up inside. Ben Wa balls, which are intended to be inserted in the anus, have strings that are meant to stay on the outside. So, be careful what you use for anal stimulation. Either ensure it is purpose-made, with a flare or string so it doesn't go all the way in, or be sure to hang onto it, and not let it disappear inside you.

If an object does go all the way in, don't worry; most will come out by using the same pushing muscle movements you use to pass faeces. However, if the object is unusually large or has sharp edges you may be stuck with a trip to the emergency department. These things are sometimes unable to be removed without a general anaesthetic. Best, if possible, not to get into this situation.

Vibrators

Most of the vibrators on the Australian market are battery-operated and are not capable of giving you a harmful shock. However, some use mains power (240 volts). A shock from mains power electricity can kill you. If the electrical connections are in good condition and the item is used in accordance with the instructions that come with it, you should have no problems. But remember, water and electricity do not mix. Never, ever use a vibrator (of any sort) anywhere near water.

Violence

The key here is to trust your instincts. If you are with someone you don't know well, always be aware that the unexpected can happen. If your gut tells you that you are unsafe, always trust it. You can work out what was truly going on later. If you are worried about a situation, get out of it.

Negotiating safe sex

When deciding what you are going to do about safe sex, weigh up the risks! Make your decisions when you are not under the influence of lust, alcohol or drugs. If you know what you want, it is easier to make sure you get it.

Negotiating safe sex can be hard. In the past most women have not felt able to ask for what they wanted sexually. What women wanted didn't really count. Women who did identify what gave them sexual pleasure, and asked for it, were considered sluts. Some women still feel uncomfortable about discussing their sexual needs openly.

To negotiate safe sex, we have to feel comfortable about stating what we want. We have to feel that we are valuable; that we deserve to be treated in a way that does not put us at risk of harm. This means that we have to step past the cultural attitudes that make raising this subject difficult.

> **CLAIRE:** *I'm an HIV counsellor. I know about safe sex. I teach people how to negotiate it! I feel so piss weak, though. When I got into my new relationship I couldn't say that I wanted to use a dam. I knew I should, but I felt too shy.*

> **SUE:** *I found it so difficult to raise the subject. I thought that Viv might think I didn't trust her, or that I thought she had a disease. I don't know what I'm going to do next time.*

> **JUDE:** *I have an 'ex' who has Hep C; she is always at me to be sure about safe sex. I've just sort of got used to it. If I don't know the person, I just have gloves, lube and a dam and just act like that's how everyone has sex. It hasn't been a problem since I started.*

The starting place is to be clear about what you want. If you don't think you'll be able to ask for it, you may consider practising with a friend. When the words have come out of your mouth on one occasion, you'll be surprised that next time it's easier to say them.

Role-playing like this can make a big difference in getting what you want.

It's a good idea to talk about safe sex before you get into a passionate situation. It's far easier to say 'I only do safe sex' in casual conversation about life in general, than it is while she is unzipping your jeans.

Another way to get the message across is to have dams, gloves and safe sex packs around. If they are lying about in your bedroom, bathroom, backpack, handbag or car glove box, she will probably see them. That makes it easier to say, 'I always use latex'.

When we are in the early stages of a relationship, we set our limits in relation to all sorts of things. It's not that difficult to let someone know where you stand on safe sex if you are already clear about it yourself. Remember, it's okay to say 'no' to any activity, even if you are already in a passionate embrace. You have the right to the kind of sex you want. You certainly have the right to reject any kind of sex you don't want.

If you know you would prefer to have safe sex, but feel it might be hard for you to ask for, give some thought to that now. What stops you being treated the way you want to be? Once you answer that question you can work out how to get what you want.

If you have chosen not to have safe sex, it is worthwhile being clear about this. You may like to consider what risks are acceptable to you.

6

Sexual Self-Intimacy: Masturbation and Fantasy

MASTURBATION

Research indicates that between 60 and 80 per cent of women masturbate at some time in their lives.[1] Two early studies in 1953 and 1973 suggested that lesbian women report masturbating more often than heterosexual women.[2] More recent work appears to confirm that about 70 per cent of lesbian women will have masturbated in the previous year while only 42 per cent of women in the total population will have done so.[3]

Most women need no instruction about masturbation. It comes naturally. A large number of self-help guides are available (see 'Resources') and many popular magazines and books discuss masturbation. In addition, there are Internet sites devoted to it.

Many women, especially older women, received messages early in life that masturbation was not acceptable.

> **MARY:** *When we were little girls my mother would occasionally pick up our hands and smell our fingers. When I was about nine I found out why. She sniffed my sister's fingers, then slapped her across the face and said 'You're not to touch yourself!' We were always getting messages about our vaginas (Mum never used that word) being dirty.*

> **JEN:** *I masturbated all through my teenage years, but I felt ashamed.*

Until the Second World War, masturbation was definitely not a subject for public discussion. Christians believed it was 'sinful'. Popular myth suggested that it would send you blind, or cause hairs to grow on the palms of your hands. Many, but not all, cultures and religions saw it as unacceptable. However, by the beginning of the postwar era, Western conservative attitudes were beginning to change. Masturbation began to be seen as an immature phase to be passed through on the way to adult sexuality.[4] By the 1970s, guilt-free masturbation began to be seen as an aspect of sexual maturity.[5] In 1974, Betty Dodson wrote *Sex for One: The Joy of Self-Loving*. She and others began running workshops to teach masturbation and the liberation of sexuality.

However, there was a long way to go before people began to talk about masturbation easily. Even today, in many social circles, it is not considered to be appropriate dinner table conversation. Nevertheless, we now live in an age of acceptance and diversity. It is the era of education and electronic communication. Technologies like the Internet make it more difficult to stifle freedom of speech. People have become more comfortable with all aspects of themselves. Betty Dodson, now over seventy, may, as she hoped, live to see the liberation of masturbation.

Lesbian women are people who have the courage to explore their sexuality and themselves. Of course, they have had a tendency to ignore the cultural taboo, and to explore their genitals.

CATH: *One of the reasons why I like masturbation so much is that it gives me the opportunity to explore myself. Literally. I find out what I like. What makes me come. And that changes from time to time. With masturbation I have expanded the sort of things that will bring me to orgasm. With fantasy and masturbation I explore new frontiers in myself. It's also private precious time alone with myself that I cherish. I will happily share my masturbation with a lover, and that's a real turn-on. But I treasure the times by myself too.*

CLAIRE: *I think I had my earliest orgasm when I was in kindergarten. I used to sit on my hand and rock back and forwards. There was a build up of tension, I would get all hot and sweaty and then there would be a muscular release. Sometimes with some shaking. I did it all over the place. Bed, school, any toilet, anywhere. In fact it's still one of the main ways that I can come quickly if I want to. It wasn't till about fourth class in primary school that I realised that it wasn't really quite the right thing to do it in public. I don't think that my teachers knew what to make of me. Looking back now, I realise how embarrassed my kindergarten teacher was. She never said anything to me about it though.*

JEN: *I go through phases. Sometimes I will masturbate four or five times a day. For days and days running. And then I may not masturbate for weeks or months. It depends on what I'm doing. If I'm working at home, and not too busy, sometimes I'll treat myself to a whole afternoon in bed. Sometimes I'll decide to set it up. I might go and hire an erotic video. Or save up a book or article. I'll often start with* *a lavender bath. I'll usually put on a perfume oil burner and light a candle. Draw the blinds and then settle in. I can end up absolutely exhausted and then sleep for a while.*

SUE: *I have different sorts of orgasms when I masturbate. Sometimes they are little ones. And some times absolutely huge. But they are sort of different to the ones I have with Viv. Sometimes it happens so fast for me. I decide I want to have sex. I move my clit in a certain way and bang.*

JUDE: *When I'm vegie shopping I keep my eye out for zucchinis of a certain size (pretty small really). I call it Italian zucs. Olive oil and a small zuc. I massage my clit with one hand and massage the zuc in and out of my bum with the other. It blows my ears off. I come in seconds.*

Masturbation is fun, there is no pressure and it is satisfying. It can be a great way to teach yourself that sex is absolutely okay, and there is no reason at all to feel guilty about it. It's the easiest way to learn about what kind of stimulation you like. This knowledge can later be brought into sexual encounters with other people.

Masturbation permits you to focus just on yourself. Your own sensations and pleasure become paramount. You are not distracted by any wish to please or pleasure a partner. It teaches you about who you are. While masturbating alone, you can be as wild or as conservative as you want. There is no-one to look on and judge. You can use any kinky object or fantasy you like. It is a way of loving yourself, nurturing yourself, celebrating yourself. It allows you to learn how to give to yourself. It also is a way of ensuring ongoing sexual satisfaction, whether or not you are in relationship. It can solve problems when two women in a relationship have different levels of sexual desire. It is the ultimate in self-sufficiency.

Masturbation may lead to improved health and emotional well-being. It releases sexual tension and consequently relaxes muscles. It is a great stress release technique.

CLAIRE: *On an occasional restless night I will masturbate until exhaustion drifts me off to sleep. Better than sleeping pills.*

If you've never had an orgasm the easiest way to start is with masturbation. What's more, if you've never had an orgasm you need to know more about yourself. If you've never done it, have a good look at yourself. Get a mirror, get a light and have a look.

If you're new to masturbation, you could consider two possible approaches. One approach would be to just start to play with yourself. In bed, in the bath or shower, while working around the house, or at any time that the thought crosses your mind. Imagine, say, in the shower, just deciding to explore yourself. Which part of your body takes your fancy? Perhaps your ears or neck, or some other non-sexual part of yourself. Let your caresses start there. And then continue wherever your fancy takes you. Light, playful exploration.

Another approach would be consciously to choose to set time aside. Choose how you would like to explore and nurture yourself. Which room would you like to be in? What sort of music do you like? Has music ever turned you on? Play that! Incense? Candles? What kind of clothes would you like to be wearing for your date with yourself? Do you want any accoutrements? Sex toys? Videos? Books? Magazines?

If you want to start with a bath or shower, you may find that you like to masturbate in or with water. Touching yourself in the shower or bath comes naturally. It's easy for the touch to become sexual. Some women find that being in water decreases their sensitivity, but many find it a turn-on. You can masturbate using a stream of water. It's easier if you have the kind of showerhead on a flexible hose, but it's not too difficult in a normal bath or shower. The trick is to position yourself in any way that gets a stream of warm water onto your clitoris, vagina, breasts or anus. In a normal bath, you may like to start with just a little water in the bottom of the bath. Be careful to get the temperature right before you start directing it onto sensitive parts of your anatomy. Lie flat on your back, with your vagina under the faucet and your legs up the end of the bath (and up the wall if there is one). You have to be a bit athletic. It's worth it for the warm tantalising sensations. It's often easy to get the water to flow onto your anus and perineum from the rear.

Also, if you have the luxury of a spa or jacuzzi, you can play with streams from the jets. Be very careful not to get high-pressure water flow inside either your vagina or anus as it can cause damage.

When you get out of the shower, if you like perfume, splash some on. Your trademark smells can come to be an erotic turn-on for you. Don't forget to sniff and enjoy yourself after a day's physical work or in the sun. The smells of your very own sweat can come to be an erotic delight.

Use your fingers to explore every part of your self. Trace out the sensuous curves of your body. Explore your armpits, your nipples, your inner thighs. Explore the curves of your backside. Stroke, cup and caress your cunt. Move from outside to inside. Move your juices all over the place. You may like to smell or taste your own juices, or rub them over your body. If you feel orgasm approaching, decrease or change the stimulation. This is a time to pleasure yourself, not just to climax. Prolong the enjoyment.

You may like to use oil or lube. Some women love the sensation, although others find that it decreases their sensitivity.

> **CLAIRE:** *I often use just a little vegetable oil. In fact I keep a small jar not far from my bed just for the purpose.*
> *Sometimes, if I'm in the mood for a bit of fun, I will oil my cunt and arsehole before I dress in the morning. I wipe up the excess oil so it doesn't stain my underwear. Just walking and working with that extra sensation of lubrication can lead to all-day pleasure, and the occasional quiet orgasm.*

Be very, very careful of perfume oils if you have sensitive skin or allergies. Vegetable oils are fine for many women. They may, however, contribute to an outbreak of 'thrush' for a few. Commercial lubes are safer.

Clothes can be erotically sensational. Choosing underwear you really like is a way of giving yourself the message that you care about and value yourself. The sensation of silk or satin against skin is delectable. Choose a few special underwear delights for yourself.

Have you ever wondered why lingerie shops manage to sell so many of those G-strings that look so uncomfortable? They are a constant erotic turn-on. No matter how conservative you look on the outside, while wearing one of these you are aware of the feel of them framing and cupping your cunt. The string rubbing your anus. Some women have no difficulty coming to orgasm simply 'riding' the fabric of their G-string.

No underwear can also be an erotic pleasure. In tight jeans the pressure from rubbing against the seams can provide sensual sensations. Just moving a little in your seat can start the stimulation over again. The feeling of a totally free cunt under a flowing skirt is another one not to be missed. Or, if you are a tease, a short, tight skirt.

It's sometimes fun to stand in front of a mirror and undress and masturbate at the same time. The sight of your own, partly clothed, erotically moving, body can lead to heightened sexual tension.

Some women can reach orgasm just from pressure on their pubic mound (see Fig. 4 in Chapter 2), or by taking hold of both lips of the vagina and moving them. Some can bring on a high state of arousal by squeezing their thighs together. These techniques are worth starting with. Even if they don't bring you to orgasm, they can be a highly erotic prelude.

Some women enjoy dildos and the many creative alternatives already discussed (see p.52). An innovative substitute found around your home may give you an inexpensive start when you're just beginning to masturbate. Look around the house and fridge. Work out what diameter suits you best. Use lots of lube. One dildo in the anus and one in the vagina at the same time can be fun. Be sure that either the dildo you insert into the anus is a properly commercially made one, or else ensure that you don't let go of it. Do not let it go all the way up inside you.

However, the majority of women do not need any fancy extras. A woman's own fingers are by far the most commonly used means of masturbating to orgasm.

For those already comfortable with masturbation, this may be a technique you haven't thought of:

JODY: *There's a method I learned recently off the Internet that's definitely worth telling you about. First of all, drip lube all over your cunt and anus and all the way in between. (I put a towel on my bed first). Then slide the index finger of your left hand into your anus and start to gently move it in and out. Then, slide the thumb of your left hand into your vagina and give yourself good stimulation. Then use your right hand to flick your clit. It's beyond belief!*

The 'G-spot' provides a source of exquisite delight for women who are investigating self-stimulation. See Appendix 2.

Masturbation is a time to honour yourself. Let yourself be totally free to seek your own pleasure. Set the scene. Allow yourself lots of time and space. Find the props that you want. If you wish, dress in clothes or lingerie to excite your sense of eroticism. Give yourself absolutely to yourself. Use whatever turns you on: fingers, carrot, cucumber, candle. Treat yourself: buy a vibrator. Be totally self-indulgent. Allow the noises that are inside you to come out. Is there a moan in there – let it out! Are there words that want to be said? Express them: whisper, speak or scream them. Fart. Burp. Whatever. Do some reading. Buy yourself erotica. Look at sexual images.

And most of all, practise!!!

When you feel comfortable masturbating by yourself, you may want to consider masturbating with a friend or lover. Let her watch you. Put on a show for her. It's a way of learning about each other.

TINA: *I get so turned on by watching Jude masturbate.*

PETA: *Sometimes we make it part of a scene. I tell her exactly what I want her to do to herself.*

FANTASY

Fantasy can stand alone as a means of providing sexual pleasure, or it can be incorporated with masturbation. If you have never been aware of the power of fantasy, try the following experiment:

> *Sit in a quiet place. Make sure you won't be disturbed. Take the phone off the hook. You are going to do a guided visualisation. Now shut your eyes. Bring into your mind's eye the image of a lemon. Imagine its colour. Its exact shape. Its size. See the marks on its skin. Imagine that you can smell its zesty fragrance. Now, in your mind, place it on a cutting board. Take a knife and slice the lemon. See, in your mind's eye, the cut flesh of the lemon. See the bursting golden particles of fruit. See the juice dripping from the surface. Pick the lemon up and bring it slowly to your lips. Take your time. In your imagination, open your mouth. Slowly bite the lemon.*

Did you feel any sensation in your mouth? Did your mouth water when, in your imagination, you bit into the lemon? Most people will experience, at the very least, increased salivation. This is because the body treats the images created by your mind as real. Imagination influences reality. A technique called creative visualisation helps people to build successful lives and careers.

Mental images can seem very real. Fantasy can be a very powerful source of sexual satisfaction. We can use our minds to create images, scenes and stories. In our daydreams we can visualise erotic situations that we would not choose to experience in real life. Fantasy can be used while masturbating to heighten sensuality. It can also be used alone without any self-touching for a high level of erotic enjoyment that needs no other addition. At least two per cent of women report the ability to reach orgasm from fantasy alone.[6] Erotic literature can be an aid to fantasy. Books, magazines and Internet sites may suggest possibilities and situations you would never have thought of.

In a world of constant change, some women like a comforting, comfortable fantasy that they can live over and over again. Women create ongoing scenarios and imaginary friends, lovers and familiar surroundings. It doesn't mean that they are out of touch with the real world. It's just a method of creating predictable pleasure.

Others constantly explore new frontiers in their mind. Some allow fantasy to teach them about hidden and confronting parts of themselves.

> **LOU:** I'm a lesbian feminist. I've been involved in the politics of gender for the last 20 years. It was very disconcerting for me when I kept having fantasies of being held still by one bloke, and fucked up the bum by another. Even as I talk about it, the sweaty smells in my imagination return to my mind. At first I reacted to myself with disgust and if the fantasy started I would consciously stop it. After being bothered by it for a couple of years I decided to just go with it and see where it went. I don't give it any meaning. Never in a million years would I actually let myself be in a situation where it could occur. I've realised that this fantasy is a huge turn-on for me. I figure it's just a part of myself. Not one that I would choose to action, but a part that exists nevertheless. I just let it be.

Women may feel comfortable or uncomfortable with the things they fantasise about. Fantasy about sexual activity which is forbidden or taboo is very prevalent. This may range from daydreaming about an unavailable partner to sexual activity involving the family cat. Erotic fantasy about rape or violent sex is common, either as recipient or the active participant. Women often feel guilty, worried or confused about their fantasies. One reaction is to try and push the thoughts away. It is important to realise that the fact that a scenario crosses your mind does not mean it is an event you would ever wish to act out. Psychologists are still debating about what fantasy means to the individual. Much research is yet to be done. For most women these types of fantasy are a way of recognising parts of themselves that may titillate, but which they do not want as part of their every day life.

Like masturbation, fantasy can be a celebration of self-sexuality. Or it can be shared. It can be tantalising (and sometimes very confronting) to disclose our fantasies to others. Sharing a fantasy can be a way of deepening trust and intimacy. Many women enjoy acting out their fantasies.

> **GINA:** *I'm really quite a shy person. But I've always had a fantasy about making love to a stranger on a train. I told Marina and we set it up. She 'picked me up' on the train to Melbourne. We played it all out and went into the loo and fucked. It was fantastic. It taught me how erotic sex can be if you have to hide the fact that it is happening. I don't think I would ever truly have done it with a stranger for real. We had a ball.*

Together, masturbation and fantasy can be a delightful source of self-intimacy for enjoyment by yourself or with a partner.

Orgasm

f you were to get all of your sexual information from the popular media, it would be easy to conclude that the only reason for having sexual activity is in order to get to orgasm. It is for some.

> **EMMA:** *Sex is a celebration for me. I absolutely love orgasm.*

> **NARELLE:** *Why bother with the whole thing if you and your girlfriend don't come?*

However, not all women feel that way.

> **PETA:** *I don't have an orgasm very often. For me orgasms are a big thing, very emotionally intense. I sometimes feel shattered after them, I feel like I open myself up so much. I like to have sex just to be intimate and feel the closeness. I don't always want the drama of an orgasm.*

Kinsey, as early as 1953, described orgasm as an 'explosive discharge of neuromuscular tension'.[1] He explained that at the peak of sexual activity, a woman may experience a very high level of muscular tension.

This tension can rise to peak intensity and then suddenly and abruptly be released. The woman is then usually in a very relaxed state.

In 1983 an English researcher described orgasm a little differently. Bancroft observed that a few seconds after a woman feels that she is about to have an orgasm there is an initial spasm of the muscles surrounding the outer third to the vagina. This is followed by a series of rhythmic contractions (usually, he says, five to eight) in number. Synchronous contractions of the anal sphincter occur in some women. He stated that uterine contractions may also occur but are less rhythmic.[2]

Investigators have considered these vaginal contractions to be the essence of the female orgasm, comparable to the rhythmic contractions that serve ejaculation in men. Other researchers and many women believe that we may experience orgasm without these vaginal contractions. This issue is still being debated.

Many women experience sexual release without repeated contractions that are noticeable to them:

> **JEN:** *Sometimes I have a 'real orgasm' by which I mean lots of shaking and muscle tension. Much more often I just get very tight (my toes curl, my legs are tight, all my bum and back muscles are tight), and then I just sigh and relax. As far as I'm concerned both are equally satisfying. I don't care if it's a 'real' orgasm or not – it feels like an orgasm to me.*

The tension and muscular contractions of the outer third of the vagina, (and sometimes of the uterus and anus) are triggered at a certain level of arousal. The whole body may be affected. Skin colour often changes to a 'rosy glow', sometimes called a 'sex flush'. The heart and breath rate increases, blood pressure rises, the breasts enlarge, nipples become erect, and muscles contract. Many women experience contractions of their back, abdomen, thighs, arms, legs, and feet. Sometimes there is one long contraction followed by release; more often there are rhythmic contractions. Women will often break out in a sweat. Some women find that they make noises or say words without planning to ('involuntary vocalisation').

Orgasms vary in intensity; the more intense ones may be felt as whole body experiences. Other orgasms that are far less intense can be equally satisfying. A feeling of calm often follows climax, and the woman's body may be very relaxed. Sometimes women want to sleep. Others just want to do it all over again. 'Pelvic congestion' (an accumulation of blood which flows to the pelvis prior to orgasm) is reversed. It is believed that this is the reason why some women find that orgasm relieves menstrual pain and cramps.

Other researchers have studied orgasm. Investigators have been able to use fibre optic and ultrasound imaging to see what really takes place in the genital tract.[3] In essence there have been few changes in our understanding of what actually happens. All of the definitions of orgasm seem to have in common a peak of tension that is then dramatically reduced.

Women's experience of orgasm is so varied that I am unable to describe a 'typical' climax. Orgasms are different for everyone:

> **JEAN:** *Orgasms are like sneezing. I can take 'em or leave 'em. I mean it. They are no big deal. I get tense. The tension dissipates. Just like sneezing. I'm not profoundly moved emotionally or spiritually. I'm just nice and relaxed. A good workout in my home gym followed by a nice warm bath feels almost as good and doesn't have all the emotional shit with it. I've come to truly believe that orgasm is over-rated. Anyway, that's how I'm living my life at the moment.*

> **NARELLE:** *It's a fantastic all over body feeling.*

> **JO:** *The first time I ever had an orgasm, I had no idea what was happening. I was standing up, she was kneeling and licking me, she had my backside in her hands and wouldn't let me move away. There was a warm rush spreading out from my cunt all up my belly and down my legs. I was shaking. I remember screaming. I thought I was going to collapse or black out. I didn't realise it was an orgasm.*

CLEO: *Funny how first orgasms stick in your mind. I still remember my first one vividly. It was in a car. She had been trying to seduce me. I was a virgin. She'd been caressing my breasts and had got my shirt open. I was wearing a very soft skirt. She caressed my thighs and buttocks through the skirt. Then she put her hand under the skirt and started touching me through my pants. She never did take them off. She eventually pulled them to one side. She stroked and moved my clit. It felt wonderful. I kept going back for more. I didn't want a relationship with her, but I liked what she did to me. At the time I was too young to know that those incredible feelings were orgasms. I worked it out later.*

Orgasm is more likely to occur when the recipient enjoys the physical sensations, and when the emotional setting is a comfortable and desirable one.[4] It is believed that female fertility is enhanced during and after orgasm.[5]

Types of orgasm

Sigmund Freud, the founder of modern psychology, was a medical practitioner who worked in Europe from 1885 to 1939. He defined two types of orgasm: 'clitoral', which resulted from clitoral stimulation, and 'vaginal', resulting from vaginal penetration. Freud argued that as a woman matured sexually she experienced a move from clitoral to vaginal orgasm. He argued that clitoral orgasms were an immature form of orgasm. It is not difficult to see why medical practitioners and sex researchers (who at that time were almost all men), had a vested interest in convincing women that orgasms resulting from having a penis in a vagina were somehow superior. Sex therapists have enjoyed arguing about this ever since. What a lot of intellectual masturbation!

After the work published in 1981 by the Federation of Feminist Women's Health Centers in the United States, it was accepted that the clitoris is an extensive organ that is intrinsically linked in structure and function with the vagina.[6] This was confirmed by Dr Helen O'Connell's recent work.[7] It is impossible to move the vagina (or to move fingers, a penis or any other object in the vagina) without providing stimulation to the clitoris. The fact is that Hite and many other researchers have found that a majority of women come to orgasm through clitoral stimulation.[8] It is no longer tenable to suggest that there are two different types of orgasm, or that one type is 'better' than another. Women have orgasms clitorally, vaginally, anally and sometimes from other non-genital touching. Some crave penetration. Others can climax just from stimulation of their nipples or breasts. Women may be aroused to orgasm without physical touch (by words, fantasy, or emotional and energetic charge).

How many orgasms?

Almost 50 years ago one of the very first studies of women's sexual function noted that approximately one-third of women never had an orgasm, and only half had orgasms regularly.[9] Despite the sexual revolution and the change in society's attitude towards sexual pleasure, large numbers of women rarely, if ever, experience orgasm. Two recent studies indicate that 23 per cent of women 'suffer from anorgasmia'.[10] 'Anorgasmia' is the medical word used to describe not being able to have an orgasm, despite appropriate sexual stimulation. The medical profession treats this as if there was something wrong. In my opinion, when a condition affects almost a quarter of the female population, it may be that it is simply a variation of normal. You have to look at why women don't experience orgasms, and whether or not they are concerned about this! This issue is discussed later in this chapter.

At the other end of the scale, some women have many orgasms. This can range from two or three orgasms to a large number:

> **SUE:** *I often have one orgasm after another. It takes hardly anything to get me triggered again. I end up absolutely exhausted, but often still don't feel sexually satisfied. It's like an itch that I don't quite succeed in scratching.*

MARGARET: *If I'm having sex every day, I can manage three or four. If I'm not having sex every day I can have more. It's pure greed. After I have had the first orgasm, all I have to do is clench my body again, focus for about ten seconds and I'm there. Second, third, clench again and I can have up to six or seven in a matter of minutes. My partner has to let the stimulus off a bit while I'm having the orgasm, then for just three or four seconds I like to be really lightly stimulated, graduating to a frantic pace. The more orgasms I've had, the harder the stimulation has to be until it gets to a point where I wouldn't try any more – I'm too exhausted. My partner's theory is that one of her orgasms equals three or four of mine. She's just jealous.*

How do women go about having orgasms?

MARGARET: *I would love to have had someone tell me exactly how to have an orgasm 30 years ago. It's hard work to know your body well enough to have orgasms. Nothing I have ever read has explained what you actually have to do inside your body to have an orgasm. I've thought about it a lot. I know it's not the same for everyone, but what I have to do is really focus in on the feeling and follow it. Really capture the feelings and pursue them. If I get distracted I fall back down the mountain and have to start again. I have to really put my body under a lot of pressure. If I relaxed I'd just lie on the bed like a corpse, and I could liken the stimulation in that state to a head massage. To do something with it, I have to put my body under tension. I sort of clench my body; so if I am on the bed with my legs spread, my toes will be clenched. There are two ways I can clench. Pushing clenching and sucking clenching. Holding on really tight. I have to do that. Having an orgasm is only partly about what my partner is doing to me. It's not so much about saying this is what I want done to me; rather, this is what I do for* *myself. If she does direct clitoral stimulation I find that really distracting and it is often a real deterrent [to orgasm]. The touch has to be slightly off to the side or above my clitoris. If there is a good rhythm I can come within a few minutes.*

LISA: *I find orgasms elusive. I don't have them whenever we have sex by any means. If I chase them it's usually a dead loss. I have to relax and just enjoy what is happening without worrying whether or not I will have an orgasm. If I worry about it, I almost always won't. When they happen they are often a surprise. Usually the feeling starts in my cunt. It feels so good. I often catch that delicious, on the edge feeling and then feel surprised. Most of the pleasure is in my cunt and also in my anus (even if it hasn't been touched I can feel the sensations there).*

Will I know if I've had an orgasm?

Maybe not!

Sandra Pertot, a sex therapist, disagrees with the widely held belief that if a woman isn't sure whether or not she's had an orgasm, then she probably hasn't.[11] She is another who compares orgasm to sneezing:

The first phase in the development of a sneeze is when the nose is stimulated in some way...the muscles around the nose start to tense.

At some point a sneeze occurs, but depending on the amount and type of stimulation, the sneeze may be a sudden explosive effort, causing people in the room to jump, or it may be a minor, quiet little effort which goes largely unnoticed. Usually, it is the type that falls somewhere in between. All of these are considered sneezes, none is considered abnormal.

Dr Pertot suggests that if you are trying to work out whether or not you have ever had an orgasm, 'do not look for the equivalent of a room-clearing sneeze'!!

Ask yourself whether you feel pleasure in your vagina, vulva, lower abdomen, anus or breasts during sexual activity. Do you notice yourself experiencing building tension and then later notice that the tension has relaxed? After sex do you feel relaxed, sleepy and satisfied? Pertot says that this is a 'mini-orgasm'.

Are orgasm and sexual satisfaction the same?

No! Orgasms may be profoundly satisfying or may leave you feeling empty.

> **CLAIRE:** *Years ago I had a one-night stand. Or more accurately I should say, 'a one-hour encounter'. The sex was explosive and incredible. After it was over I felt dirty, used and empty. It was an experience, I guess. I'd always fantasised about something like that. I'm not sorry I did it, but it's not something I'd be tearing out to do again. Since then I've chosen to have sex only with people I know and want to be with.*

For many lesbian women it's not just the orgasm that counts. It's the way in which they are connecting with another person. There is often an element of opening heart and soul that goes along with allowing another person intimate access to your body.

Lots of women, on the other hand, are delighted to have sex purely to luxuriate in the physical sensations. Some enjoy being able to have sexual contact briefly, and then move on to whatever occupies their lives next.

> **NARELLE:** *Recreational sex can be like sport, you practise and just get better. You don't always need the emotional involvement.*

Large numbers of people now believe that there is no right or wrong about sexual satisfaction unless it is non-consensual or hurts another person.

The absent orgasm

Western culture is a goal-orientated, achievement-driven society. Orgasm, is, in our culture, portrayed as the goal of sex.

This is only one of the possibilities. Our culture could have chosen physical pleasure as the goal, or joy, or delight in connection with another human being.

Due to our present cultural attitudes, women who don't have orgasms sometimes feel like failures. But remember, in Victorian England, women who didn't have orgasms were regarded as normal and virtuous. Women who did have orgasms were regarded by 'nice' people as lustful and amoral! In those days 'good' women did not seek pleasures of the flesh!

It is important to look at why women don't have orgasms. There are many reasons. A woman's family and religious background may influence whether she feels relaxed and able to enjoy her sexuality. Even the most conservative researchers agree that psychological and emotional factors determine what will happen.[12] If a woman feels relaxed, happy and loved she is more likely to have an orgasm than if she feels unsafe, not respected, betrayed or used.

This is not universally true. Some describe being turned on to orgasm by people that they dislike profoundly. For many, the thrill of a casual encounter may lead to heightened pleasure and sexual intensity. However, lots of women are unable to have orgasms unless they have an emotional connection with their sexual partner. Even a small issue causing relationship conflict can take away the possibility of orgasm. For these women, issues causing disharmony have to be resolved before sex.

Orgasm issues may have to do with trust and surrender. They may also have to do with how you feel about the relationship.

It is important to consider the function of orgasm. Early thinkers suggested that orgasms exist in order to make sex enjoyable, so that humans will have a reason to seek sex and therefore procreate the species. However, if that were the case, you wouldn't be able to masturbate yourself to orgasm. Just think – if someone else tickles you, the sensation may be exquisite or unbearable. But if you tickle yourself, nothing happens. Your neurological circuits know that you are providing the stimulation and tickling has no effect. The human organism is sufficiently complex to distinguish between the two. We could have been set up with an orgasmic system that only fires if the stimulus is from another person (or from a person of the opposite sex, if homophobes are right). But we weren't! We were set up with a sexual neurology that permits and provides pleasure from both self-stimulation and couple sex (with partners of both genders).

It's my theory that the purpose of orgasm is for release of tension, for pleasure and just for fun. I would take this theory a bit further and say that the pleasure can be either purely in the body, or can also include emotional, intellectual and spiritual aspects. What happens depends on the type of person you are.

Some people are very physical. They live their lives through the experience of the body. Others are 'thinkers'. The most important thing for them is what goes on in their minds. They are often very rational. They make their decisions and choices after thinking things through. Others are 'feelers'. Their most important reality is the one they sense emotionally. They relate to the world through their own feelings and responding to the feelings of others. Yet others find the spiritual dimension the most meaningful aspect of existence. We are all influenced by each of these factors, but often, one will tend to dominate.

The way you experience enjoyment, and the nature of the pleasure you desire, will depend on the sort of person you are. For many women, sexual intimacy and orgasm are the culmination of a relationship. Emotional, intellectual and spiritual intimacies are the base on which physical intimacy and orgasm rest. However, for countless numbers of other women, sex is 'just good fun'. These women can experience pleasure in their bodies without necessarily involving their hearts, spirits and minds. There is no right or wrong in this issue. It is a matter of working out who you are and what you want, and honouring that.

It is possible that if a woman is not having orgasms, there may be some element of contact in the body, mind, emotional, or spiritual matrix that is not present in the sexual connection for her. I would offer the suggestion that this is okay! Our partners are not necessarily put on earth to meet us in every physical, mental, emotional and spiritual aspect of ourselves. We can still have perfectly good and very enjoyable sex with them! It may be that it is up to us to get some of our needs met by another means.

It is also possible that if a woman is not having orgasms, the reason lies entirely within her, and does not lie in the nature of the sexual connection at all. She may be simply too tired, her concerns may not be sexual at that moment, she may have had a previous difficult sexual experience that is not yet resolved, or her family upbringing may have conditioned her into believing that sexual pleasure is wrong.

The absence of orgasms is only a problem if you want to have them and can't.

Can I learn to have an orgasm?

Yes, most probably you can. Many women need to learn how to have orgasms because our culture has trained them not to enjoy sex (see the next chapter).

The most important thing about orgasm is not to get hung up on it. Treat it as you would treat a butterfly; appreciate it if it comes by!

8

Difficulty With Sex

The existing studies of lesbian sexuality are inadequate. There is no satisfactory evaluation of the sexual problems experienced by lesbian women. However, from the information available, overall sexual satisfaction seems high.[1]

GETTING THE BASICS RIGHT

If you are having difficulty enjoying sex, it is important to consider that sometimes really simple issues can be part of the problem. Sexual pleasure can be impaired by discomfort, therefore the physical environment is important, and can make or break an encounter. Ensuring that you are comfortable in your physical surroundings may sometimes solve problems.

> **CLAIRE:** *The best thing we ever did was move out of the house we were sharing. I always worried that the woman who had the bedroom next to ours could hear everything we did, every noise we made. I was completely unable to relax.*

I couldn't focus my attention on anything except awareness of every movement or moan either of us made.

Secure the level of privacy you need. For some women, the thought that they might be seen or heard adds a little spice to the encounter. Others are frozen both emotionally and physically. If your environment makes obtaining privacy difficult, be inventive. Take advantage of occasions when other household members are out. If you have children, you may want to plan some childfree time.

Ensure that you are comfortable in your surroundings. It's for your pleasure. It's important to go after what you want.

> **JULES:** *It got to the point where I didn't feel like having sex. Lisa always wanted to have all the blankets off when she went down on me. The room was like a bloody icebox! Also, I was uncomfortable feeling that naked. I felt like a 'wuss'. I didn't say anything for ages. In the end I told her what the problem was. We went out and bought a good heater. Mostly I keep my shirt on now so I don't feel like I'm laid out like a piece of meat. It's made a huge difference.*

Also, take whatever steps you need to be comfortable in yourself. Some women love the smells and tastes of unwashed woman-flesh. They enjoy their own body odour and those of others. Other women are very uncomfortable with sexual activity if they are unshowered. Taking time to bathe can transform a sexual experience by dissolving self-consciousness. There may be other particular or special things you need so that you can feel relaxed and at ease. Ensuring that your desires are met in relation to the preliminaries will set the scene for a nurturing sexual encounter.

PROBLEMS WITH DESIRE

If a lesbian woman or couple wants to talk about sexual difficulties, the most likely thing to be discussed will be issues of desire.[2] Many, many women go through periods where they just don't feel like having sex. Lack of desire is the most common sexual problem for all women (lesbian and heterosexual). Sexual desire is also called 'libido'; lack of desire may be referred to as 'low libido'.

Is it really low libido?

Some health professionals treat lack of desire as if it is a disorder. There is even a psychiatric diagnosis: 'Hypoactive Sexual Desire Disorder'.[3] However, low sexual desire is so common in women that it seems to me that it is usually a variation of normal, and is not pathological. Popular culture bombards us with sexual imagery. We are exposed to constant updates on the sexual pairings of public figures. The media's 'ideal' woman is beautiful and sexually passionate. What nonsense! The average woman has a partner, may have children, a dog to feed, the shopping to do, a job, and household or social responsibilities. She has many more concerns than what might go on between the sheets at night. She may be passionately interested in music, cooking, surfing or Egyptian art. But the demands of life mean that these things have to take a back seat, often for very long periods of time. The same goes for sex!

The mundane, everyday necessity to survive life sometimes means that sexual pleasure is not a high priority. Major life stressors may affect libido profoundly.

> **FIONA:** *In my first year as an intern I was continually stressed. I was not sure that I could do the job. I loved my partner but often did not want to make love. I was anxious about getting enough sleep, and anxious generally. It blew our sex life out the window.*

> **LAURA:** *Last year we moved three times. I had a new job. My partner was out of work for a while and her mother, who we both loved, died. Sex just didn't happen at all for about eighteen months. At first I thought there was something wrong and that we were growing apart. After talking to a counsellor together we realised it was just everything that had happened to us.*

Lack of desire may be simply the result of being overtired and over-committed. If you simply don't feel interested in sex, don't worry. Vast numbers of women feel like you. And they are normal!

Desire and the nature of lesbian relationships

The dominant culture defines sex as 'penis in vagina'. Within lesbian relationships, certain activities can come to be defined as sex. These may include finger to vulva, finger in vagina, mouth to vagina, and vaginal or anal penetration with toys or dildoes.

In a television episode of 'Sex in the City', a woman playing the role of a lesbian states: 'If you don't eat pussy, honey, you're not a dyke'. This is not true!

There is no real reason why any such definitions make sense. Once you decide that the definition of sex goes beyond the activity necessary for reproduction (and this is essential if you believe that what lesbians do is sex), then it's all about pleasure. Whatever intimate activities give you pleasure may be defined as sexual.

Sometimes women find that their need for intimacy is met through cuddling and caressing. This is one of the ways in which lesbian relationships differ from heterosexual ones. It is thought that the majority of women find emotional closeness and non-genital caresses important.[4] In contrast, many men feel that closeness is attained through sexual contact.[5] They will therefore seek genital sexual activity. In lesbian relationships, however, both women may seek non-genital intimacy. If intimacy needs are satisfied by snuggling, caresses and cuddling, long periods may pass when neither partner initiates (or feels like) touching the other's genitals.

The Australian lesbian psychotherapist and songwriter, Georgia Carr, performs her own beautiful song 'High Romance'. In it she gently jokes about the relatively low importance of reaching a climax to many lesbians. The chorus tells a common story:

> High Romance, let's give it whirl,
> let's fill the old bathtub,
> throw in some Epsom salts, some rose and lavender oil,
> And we can slip into bed between the sun-dried sheets, fluff
> up the pillows and snuggle up tight,
> And if we fall asleep because we're too damn tired, we're on
> a promise for tomorrow night…

And there's the old lesbian joke:

> Q: When lesbians have been together for five years, how
> often do they have sex?
> A: What's sex?

Psychologists have suggested theories to explain this difference between lesbian and heterosexual relationships. The essential nature of lesbian relationships has been described by words like 'fusion' and 'merger'. It is suggested that lesbian couples are closer, more interdependent and spend more time together than heterosexual couples.[6] If genital sexual activity reflects an impetus to 'merge' for the moment, couples who are already merged may feel less drive for this type of union.[7]

Why is low desire a problem?

Is it because you yourself would like to have sex more often? Or is it because you want to please your partner or meet society's image of what a sexual person should be like?

MARIE: *If it wasn't for Annie, I wouldn't care if we never had sex. I'm just not interested at the moment. I make love with her because I don't want her to think I don't love her. I hate to see how disappointed she is when I don't want to.*

MELANIE: *I feel like a weirdo in my circle of friends. What interests them is who is doing what to whom, and how. I don't feel like being sexual. To be honest, I'm going through a bit of a spiritual time and I just want to be with myself on that. But sometimes I feel such a misfit that I think I should do something about myself.*

It's worth taking time to work out how you really feel. If you realise that you don't mind how you are, but that your low desire is only a problem for you because of your partner or someone else, then remember: their sexual desire is their problem. You are not on this planet to fix it for them. (See 'Desire Discrepancies', p. 112.)

Medical causes of low desire

Reduced sexual desire is not commonly caused by medical disorders. However, there are some conditions that should be considered.

Depression may be the cause of reduced or absent sexual desire. This is a treatable condition, and can be addressed by a health professional. Medication can be very effective in relieving symptoms. However, some anti-depressant medications are themselves the source of reduced desire.

Medications used to treat high blood pressure can result in reduced or absent desire. Problems may also be caused by steroids, and by medicines used to treat ulcers, anxiety, epilepsy and psychiatric illness. If you are on any medication and notice a decrease in sexual appetite that is out of character for you, it is important to discuss this with the person who prescribed the treatment.

Menopause may be associated with decreased sexual interest. However, less than 20 per cent of women notice a significant decline in libido and at least half do not notice any diminished interest.[8] It has been demonstrated that decreasing oestrogen levels are not the cause of reduced libido.[9] However, androgen deficiency does seem to have an impact. Small doses of testosterone to supplement those naturally produced by the body may be helpful if this is found to be the problem.[10]

Poor general health, or the existence of a major physical illness, may cause sexual desire to disappear. If lack of interest is new and unusual for you, a health check-up may be indicated.

If sexual activity has been painful on several occasions (see p. 116), fear can decrease libido. It is important to have pain assessed by a health professional. If you have difficulty with orgasm, sometimes repeated disappointment can mean that there is no desire to 'try again'. Sexual urges may disappear. If reduced libido is due to problems around orgasm, please see pp 121–125.

Drugs and alcohol

Overuse of alcohol, marijuana, cocaine, 'speed' (amphetamines), 'benzos' (benzodiazepines) and other sedatives, heroin, other narcotics and anabolic steroids can result in a lack of interest in sexual activity. If you think your problem with desire might be related to drug use, it is time to think about what is most important to you.

> **MARGARET:** *Drugs make it more difficult. I find that if I've taken drugs, particularly ecstasy, it's damn near impossible to have an orgasm. I don't think you should necessarily try and fuck on drugs. E is definitely not a fuck drug. You pursue and pursue orgasm and you just can't have one. I take E if I want to go out and dance all night, but not if I know I want to fuck.*

Sexual desire may be permanently impaired by long-term drug use. However, when the drug use ceases, desire will usually slowly return.

Is it you, your partner, or the way you relate?

Desire is so complex that it can be very difficult to work out where the problem lies. It may be a mix of factors. The make-up of your personality, your past experiences, the way you are triggered by your present partner and the circumstances of your relationship, may all combine to have an effect.

If you have a level of desire that is lower than you would like, it may be helpful consider a few questions:

- What activities do you include when you think about sex?
- At this moment, do you feel like sex? Do you feel like intimacy? What is the difference?
- If you don't feel like sex, is this alright with you? (If it is not, what stops it from being alright?)
- Have you ever felt like sex?
- Has there ever been a time in the past when you felt more like sex?

If you have low desire and feel okay about it, there is no problem at all. If, however, you would like to change your low desire, take heart. It may well be possible. You may have to take a careful look within yourself, at your partner, and at your relationship.

First of all, check out what is going on within you. After reading the first part of this chapter, I'm sure you will have already asked yourself: 'Am I getting enough sleep?' 'Am I totally overwhelmed by life's stressors?' These basic issues need to be addressed first. Sexual drive springs from the overflow of well-being in your life. There has to be a certain level of fundamental ease and sufficiency before it can exist. So attend to these essentials initially.

It's me, I know it's me

When you look within yourself, are you simply uninterested in sex? Or do you feel a sense of wanting to avoid it? Issues in the past contribute to who you are now. Previous psychological trauma can leave lasting scars. Women who have experienced past ill treatment may feel panic, rage, revulsion or a range of other feelings. However, these are often strong feelings, not simply lack of interest. If you have a suspicion that desire problems may have their roots in previous abuse, it would be worth considering taking steps to find a health professional you trust and discussing it with them (see 'Resources', p. 239).

Dealing with old pain may take some time. The decision to do so may be difficult to make. It may feel scary and confronting, but it's worth it! Whether we know it or not, many of our present reactions and decisions are influenced by our history. One of the things a counsellor can do is provide safety and support while we venture into the scary and difficult parts of our past. Looking into these problems brings awareness, and it becomes possible to see why present patterns of behaviour occur. Then we can make different choices. By acknowledging what has happened, many women are able to move beyond the pain. Choosing not to face things takes a lot of energy. It also means you are hiding parts of you from yourself and the world. Choosing to face the hidden wounds allows you access to all of yourself. Often this means you find out about strength and capability you didn't know you had. Many women have taken this path to walk into their futures empowered!

Sex is about having someone inside your physical boundaries. Look at what we do when we make love: her tongue may be in your mouth. Her fingers may be in your vagina. She is literally inside you. It is my belief that for lots of women, it is very difficult to have someone inside your physical boundaries without also letting them inside your emotional and spiritual boundaries. Plainly, desire issues may be boundary issues.

> **CLAIRE:** *I've had relationships where I've really felt overwhelmed by the other person. I just didn't stand up for myself. For a very long time I haven't felt like sex at all. I know a big part of it is that I'm afraid that if I have sex with someone, then I won't be able to defend myself from them. That is what happened last time. It was my fault, of course. I allowed it to happen. She was just being herself. And it really*

*feels clear to me that it's not that I don't trust other women.
It's that I don't trust myself to act in my own best interests
once I'm in a relationship. And I know that if I have sex,
then I always end up in a relationship. Until I feel certain
that I can do better at this I want to stay celibate. It's not
much of an issue. The sexual urge just isn't there. At an
absolute gut level I'm so terrified around this. Sooner or later
I guess I'd better get some counselling.*

Women who have difficulty identifying and maintaining their
boundaries may initially permit a great deal of closeness. They then
notice that this is more than they are comfortable with. In reaction to
this, they may throw up defences, retreat, and notice a diminution in
sexual desire. It takes time and maturity to learn the skill of creating
comfortable boundaries and also permitting appropriate intimacy.

Sometimes women feel so unhappy with who they are that they are
not able to expose themselves to another person. Connection with
others becomes difficult. Sexual desire dies. These feelings may spring
from issues around body image or disability. There may not be a
physical issue behind the problem. Self-hatred or low self-esteem can
spring from a myriad of sources: too tall, too fat, breasts too big (or
small), a mastectomy, too old (or too young), not smart enough, too
intellectual, too strong, too yuppie, too working-class, too butch, too
femme, the wrong skin colour – there is no end to the things which
women can find to be profoundly uncomfortable about. Usually, it is
not just one particular issue. There will often be several. If it seems that
feelings about your self-image are preventing you from fully
experiencing your sexual desire, it is time to become self-nurturing.

Issues may be so deep-seated that they can only be addressed in
counselling or psychotherapy. However, often self-help groups can be
life-changing.

Sometimes lesbian women feel guilty about their sexual feelings.
Guilt may inhibit the sex drive of all people: women and men, gay and
straight. The source of guilt about sex is usually found in the attitudes
that we absorbed while growing up.

We have grown into adults and have now formed our own views and values. However, the impact of our parents, teachers and other powerful people in our childhood and adolescence can be very difficult to escape. Their continuing influence may be very subtle. It can be very difficult for adults to shake off these early influences.

Religions have had the effect of making people feel guilty about sexual thoughts and activities for centuries. Many religious authorities condemn every sexual activity except that which occurs within heterosexual marriage. Some religions even dictate the positions acceptable for sexual congress and the appropriate thoughts that a person should be having at the time! Guilt is a tool effectively utilised by many religious systems to ensure that people conform. Religions are particularly vicious in their condemnation of homosexuality. Large numbers of lesbian women have struggled with guilt arising from their religious backgrounds. Some women feel that spirituality is an essential part of their nature. For such women, a conservative religious childhood, in addition to the realisation of lesbian identity, may lead to internal conflict that can stifle sexual desire.

Recognition that spirituality and religion are distinct and separate can release us from the chains of religious dogma. There are people and organisations that seek spiritual truth and worship without the need for condemnation. Contact with these souls can help heal profound wounds caused by those who censure and castigate (see 'Resources', p. 258).

Until the late twentieth century, homosexual sexuality was not acceptable in our culture. Many women have struggled to accept their sexual orientation. If this is a problem for you, it may help to know you are not alone. Even those of us who are out, proud and feel well adjusted are occasionally confronted by our own internalised homophobia (see p. 10). We live in a culture that until very recently condemned us. Even though things are changing, it is not surprising that we may sometimes feel guilt about our lesbian sexual desire. As a result women may consciously or unconsciously repress their sexual feelings. This results in decreased sexual drive.

All people have aspects of themselves that cause them some kind of conflict. If you have decided that you identify yourself as lesbian, and you are experiencing conflict or guilt, counselling may be a useful option to consider. Accepting yourself as an adult whose views and values are the only valid base from which to live your life may sometimes be a starting place. Moving gently towards accepting and loving yourself will defuse issues of guilt and conflict in time. Self-education, books and support groups may help. JoAnn Loulan[11] has written an excellent chapter on this subject. She provides useful exercises to assist in letting go of guilt and homophobia.

The Coalition of Activist Lesbians has, in conjunction with the NSW Department for Women, produced a three-part resource package called 'Out For Action: Enhancing Lesbian Lives' (see 'Resources', p. 255). This package is for use in small groups and workshops. The aim of the kit is 'to assist "out" lesbians to support new and emerging lesbians of all ages'. Taking part in such a lesbian-focused workshop run by women who have 'been there, doing that' goes a long way towards defusing guilt and internalised homophobia.

It is important to realise that desire may be influenced as much by what is happening outside us as by our internal state of being. If you have had a long hard look at yourself and still don't know why there is no drive, turn your mind to the way in which you and your partner relate.

Partnership issues

Are there things in this area that need addressing? If relationship disharmony exists, it can have a big impact on sexual desire. As a couple, you will need to consider setting time aside to sort the issues out.

It may also be important to ask yourself whether this relationship is the right place for you to be. In the relationship, do you feel affirmed and nurtured? Do you feel respected? Do you have the space to be who you really are? Or do you feel that you are overruled, and your limits and boundaries are invaded? What sort of a person are you in this relationship? Does it bring out aspects of your personality that you like and respect? Do you like the way you feel when you are together?

Are you really attracted to her, or are you in this relationship for some other reason? If you feel deep discomfort around any of these questions, you need time and space to let the answers emerge. It may not be possible to solve sexual difficulties in the face of serious, persistent relationship dissonance.

Women who feel overly merged with their partner may sometimes seek emotional and physical space by resisting sexual connection. This may occur at a conscious level. It may also occur far below the level of consciousness, so that you are not aware what is happening. If you do not feel respected, or if you feel that your limits and boundaries are continually being breached, it may be difficult or impossible to open yourself up for sexual contact. Libido may be reduced or absent. Instead, your defences will be in place.

Desire will probably not arise until these issues have been addressed.

Assertiveness training may assist you to get what you want. There are short courses that teach simple, learnable strategies, giving women tools that empower them to identify, ask for and obtain the things that are important to them. Many women's health centres and adult education organisations offer this training. If sexual feelings have been smothered by a relationship that is overclose, negotiating more individual space may allow sexual feelings to grow.

If the way you and your partner relate to each other has led to desire problems, then it is important to talk about it. Acknowledge that the two of you have an issue that needs attention and set time aside. It's best to talk when neither of you is tired or sexually aroused. If you are both busy people, it may be that you need to agree on a time and place. It's wise to pick a place where you do not usually have sex. If you mostly have sex in the bedroom, then have this conversation in the lounge. The setting will help give you both a bit of psychological distance from the issue. It may take several sessions. Try and ensure that there will be no interruptions. Take the phone off the hook. You need to have the courage to honestly allow your feelings to be known. This may feel frightening, but what have you got to lose? Even more importantly, you also need to listen to each other. Just give the issue space. Solutions may often clearly present themselves. If they do not, each of you may take the time to write down three possible ways to resolve the problem. Make sure that what you write would suit you! Then share what you have written with each other. If a workable answer does not seem obvious, don't despair. Give the matter time. Agree on another time to talk in a week or so, and repeat the process. Just living with the new knowledge that you have about yourself and your partner will often suggest answers.

There are several excellent books that address issues of difficulty in lesbian relationships (see 'Resources'). Some provide exercises you can work through together. It may also be worth considering relationship counselling.

Desire discrepancy

Difficulties may arise if you are in a relationship with someone who wants sex more frequently than you do.

> **CLEO:** *When Steph and I were first in the relationship we delighted in sex with each other. But there came a point when I was tired (I was working long hours) and didn't want to have sex as often as she did. Or maybe I just have a lower sex drive than her. Then we got into a 'vicious cycle'; I knew she wanted more sex than we were having, but she didn't pressure me (much). I felt guilty, but also, because of the unspoken pressure, something inside me died. I went off sex altogether. She decided I must have been abused in the past (I wasn't). It was just the unstated pressure. I froze. Looking back, I realise now that it was a sort of silent power struggle. When she ended our relationship she said it was because of other issues, but I believe that this was probably the main one. If I were to have a chance to do it over again, I would make sure it was all brought right out into the open.*

Desire discrepancy is the couple's problem. Each woman represents a different aspect of the situation. Each of you must negotiate what you want. Be careful how you balance your needs against the needs of the relationship. It is really important to remember that it is not your job to solve your partner's problems. You are not responsible for meeting her sexual needs.

> **JEN:** *Karen and I had different sex drives. Thank god we were able to talk about it. Usually, if I felt sexual I masturbated. Sometimes by myself, sometimes with Karen watching or stroking me. There would be times when it would turn her on and we would make love. Sometimes it would make her feel the need to get away into her own space, so she would. Most of the time, I would tell her when I felt sexual. Occasionally she would offer me a massage. We both really had to sort out when we wanted sex, and when what we wanted was intimacy.*

If your partner wants to have her sexual urges met, both she and the two of you as a couple could think about how this might be achieved. How would she meet her sexual needs if you were not around?

If you are the one who wants to have sex when your partner doesn't, would dancing go some way towards meeting the need? What about masturbation? Exercise? Having a massage? Just choosing to let it pass? Let's face it, we don't act on every sexual urge we have. Is this an occasion when what you want is intimacy? Could she meet you halfway by offering to swap non-sexual stroking? A foot massage? A head massage? A facial? Ultimately, it's your need. It's up to you to sort out what to do about it without imposing on her.

> **SARAH:** *I have to feel sufficiently comfortable with myself to be able to participate fully in a relationship. It's not a question of my needs versus the relationship needs; it's about achieving a balance.*

These issues go to the core of attitudes about sex and relationship. Some lesbian women avoid the problem of desire discrepancy by never entering a monogamous relationship. Women who have very high libidos may choose to remain footloose and fancy-free. Some choose to have a primary relationship with differing agreements about sex outside the main relationship. One couple has agreed that they may each have sex outside the relationship, but will always have safe sex and will never spend the night away from home. Another couple has agreed that it is okay to have sex outside the primary relationship but neither wishes to know what the other is doing. There are many different types of agreement that women feel comfortable with.

However, by far the majority of lesbian women are in monogamous relationships.[12] We will almost all experience desire discrepancy at some point. Many of us have found ways of dealing with it. The person with the higher libido will not always get what they want. The person with the lower desire may find it useful to remember the sexual response cycle (see p. 30). JoAnn Loulan suggests that the first stage in the sexual response cycle is willingness.[13] This may mean an active choice to be available for sex, even if you don't really feel like it. Would it feel okay to you to make an agreement to set time aside for sex, even when you don't think there are any sexual urges in you? You may not be prepared to have genital touching. There may be other sexual practices that you don't want. But would you be prepared to create ambience and conditions that you both like, so that sexual intimacy can happen anyway?

Or, as a couple, are you both prepared just to let sex lie dormant for a while?

> **SARAH:** *If sex isn't happening, but love and attraction are still strong, we remain optimistic that sex will happen again. It's a very basic thing, but it buys space. It creates an intimate safety in those non-sexual times. We have been through enormous things as a couple. But we sort of say, 'Hey, it's okay, it will happen again when there's space in our lives again'. And it does.*

At the end, you have to make the decision that is best for you. If you are clear that you don't want sex, then it may be important to find ways to bolster your boundaries against repeated incoming messages from society generally and your partner in particular, that you 'should' be more sexual. These messages may be very subtle. A partner's facial expression and body language expressing disappointment may have a powerful impact.

When you work out what you truly feel, it could be the right thing for you to compromise and shift position. However, if this results in sexual activity that is deeply unwanted, the cost may be too high. Resentment (or suppressed anger) towards a partner may be destructive. Turned inwards, it affects the way you feel about yourself. Either way, it may end in destroying the relationship. This is one of those things where being true to yourself is really important.

If you feel unable to change things at present, it helps to remember that lack of drive is usually cyclic! You will, almost certainly, feel like having sex again.

Broader desire issues

If desire discrepancy in your relationship feels overwhelming, it may be useful to remember that desire fits into a broader context. All human relationships experience disparate desire all the time: I want a 'Big Mac', you want a vegetarian lentil burger. We sort it out. It's part of life. Not a big deal. Desire discrepancy is nothing special – it's part of mundane day-to-day living.[14]

Desire is also part of the spiritual world. In Buddhism, all suffering is thought to arise from desire, attachment or craving.[15] There's some truth in that. Notice how much angst and misery occur when we do not get what we want (sexually and in all other ways). Imagine what it would be like if you could just let go and enjoy every aspect of whatever happens without any preconceived notions of what ought to be taking place. Lives (and sex lives) would change dramatically. Many systems of philosophy and spirituality attempt to place desire in context and suggest ways of dealing with it. Working out what you want, how to get it, and how to react if your desires are not met is one of the tasks of being human.

Excessive libido

Interestingly, libido considered 'too low' attracts a specified psychiatric diagnosis. Sexual desire which is unpleasantly strong or frequent for the person who has it does not. Nevertheless, women sometimes recognise that their sex drive is uncomfortable for them. 'Sexual addiction' is the behaviour of seeking sexual activity when the result will be damaging to your physical or mental well-being. There are a number of different underlying causes. A very common cause is a craving for cuddles and intimacy. Women frequently initiate sex excessively in order to feel wanted.

> **LISA:** *I used to have sex all the time because it was the only way I ever felt loved.*

Rarely, 'a woman is desperately trying to learn to orgasm, and is badgering her partner to practice at every opportunity'.[16] More often, the impetus may be simply to create a thrill or high similar to that experienced by people who choose drugs or alcohol instead. Women who have a problem with sexual addiction will compulsively have sex that threatens relationships, friendships, employment and their own self-respect. As with substance addiction, the first step to dealing with sexual addiction is to admit that there is a problem (see 'Resources').

PAIN OR DISCOMFORT

Lubrication

You may have very adequate sexual desire but nevertheless find that you do not experience the arousal response. You are turned on, but there is little swelling of the vagina and vulva. The flow of vaginal juices may be minimal. Women may experience this as a frequent event or just a passing phase. It is another very common complaint made by both lesbian and heterosexual women. Happily, the solution is not far away. Reach for the tube of lube! Buy it in bulk!!

There some conditions associated with the problem. Menopause and reduction in oestrogen levels may be associated with vaginal dryness. Lactation (breastfeeding an infant) may be a cause. Some of the medications and medical conditions referred to on p. 104 may also interfere with the body's normal function.

Often there is no obvious reason for absent lubrication. Don't think it means you aren't turned on: trust your feelings. If you are the partner, don't feel rejected, don't think she's not attracted to you. Trust what she whispers in your ear, and how the rest of her body responds to you.

Don't worry about it. It's common, and usually no cause is ever found. Compensate with saliva and lube and have fun.

Clitoral pain

Clitoral pain is one of those things that you don't hear much about. It is not uncommon. The most usual cause is friction. The clitoris is a delicate organ, comprised of tender tissues and multiple nerve endings. The very sensitivity that gives exquisite pleasure to some of us means that even gentle manipulation can be painful for others. Some women find direct touch on the glans (or tip) or the clitoris distressing and unpleasant. If clitoral pain is a problem, change what you are doing. Indirect clitoral stimulation by moving the whole pubic mound, or by moving the clitoris from inside the vagina, may be more pleasurable. Using the tongue and lots of saliva to stimulate the area surrounding the clitoris, rather than the clitoris itself may be more acceptable than the touch of a finger or dildo. New clitoral pain, not attributable to stimulation, in a woman who doesn't usually experience it is an indication for a health check. Infection needs to be excluded.

dical conditions

Vaginal or vulval pain while having sex may be due to vaginal or urinary tract infection. Vaginal scar tissue, endometriosis, adhesions, fibroids and other gynaecological conditions can be a cause. If you have had sex without difficulty in the past, and develop pain or discomfort, the first thing to do is get a sexual health check-up.

Haemorrhoids may make anal sex painful or impossible. Other physical conditions, such as arthritis, back injures and various abdominal problems, may make sex painful. If you have any of these conditions, you may have to get inventive. It doesn't mean you can't have sex. It just means you have to modify what you can do to pleasure each other.

Pain deep within the pelvis on penetration may simply be due to unskilful thrusting with a vibrator, dildo or finger. It may also be caused by torn ligaments after childbirth or other trauma to the genital tract. However, persistent deep pain is always an indication for a health check. It can be caused by infection, endometriosis, tumours, and by other serious conditions that may be treatable.

Vaginismus

Vaginismus is pain when the vagina is penetrated. Some women have pain when penetration is even attempted. 'Primary vaginismus' is when a woman has never had vaginal penetration. 'Secondary vaginismus' is when a woman has experienced vaginal penetration in the past without difficulty. Vaginismus is caused by spasm of the vaginal muscles. It may be so severe that a woman may have difficulty using tampons. It is believed that it is always due to fear either of sex or of being hurt.

Primary vaginismus may occur after physical or sexual abuse, difficult past sexual experiences or for many other emotional reasons, including that the woman believes her sexual activity is morally wrong. It could possibly be triggered by frightening or unskilful gynaecological examinations.

A vaginal infection which caused pain but has now resolved after treatment, can set up a vicious cycle where there is a part of a woman's mind that expects sex to hurt, so she tightens up. Because she is tight, penetration hurts, and the cycle continues.

However, it seems that vaginismus can occur if a woman at a deep psychological level, for whatever reason, does not want to be sexual with her partner, or is angry with her partner.

When women have vaginal pain due to vaginismus, they may already be aware of what has triggered it for them. They may be well aware of an event that took place, and yet be unable to relax their vaginal muscles.

Other women have no idea what may have triggered the condition and may reject the idea that it is caused by fear. Nevertheless, if these women are given sedative medications or placed under an anaesthetic for examination to ensure that there is no physical problem, in almost all cases their vaginas will become elastic and penetration easily takes place. This makes it clear that what is going on is in some way related to the way the mind is affecting the body.

Some women do not like penetration and have no wish to change this. They may like lesbian sex because one can have an active lesbian sex life, and still choose not to have any penetration of any sort, ever.

Vaginismus can be treated, and the success rate is very high. However, as most of us know, simply telling ourselves to relax only works sometimes. Usually the first step is to become familiar with the way your own body works, to become more educated about sex generally, and to explore what you would like to take place in your sex life. The next step (if you haven't already done so) is to explore your own genitals, and see what, if anything, you can put in your vagina.

Special 'trainers' called 'Amielle trainers' exist. They are like dildos with handles. They come in graded sizes. However, they are expensive, and not easy to get hold of. The idea is to find out what you are comfortable with, and to increase this, until you are happy that you can get what you want in your vagina. You can use any object you choose. Will a lubricated matchstick slide in and out? If yes, will a string bean or biro, which has been lubricated, fit? Experiment with very slim objects and find what you can slide in and out. Will your littlest finger fit? Will a tampon or index finger? Sex shops sell dildos and vibrators in sizes ranging from very slim to huge. As you become comfortable with objects that are the size you want to accept, you can experiment with allowing your partner to penetrate you. This must be under your control. You should have an agreement that your partner will stop immediately when you say to.

At some point, it is often useful to explore (with a therapist or other person you feel comfortable with) where the fears or feelings that cause the muscle spasm may be based. It is not necessary to do this to solve the problem, though. Sometimes this exploration is best left until after you are comfortable. For other women, realising where the problem originates may help you let it go. It may, however, make no difference at all.

Pain when no cause is found

'Dyspareunia' is painful intercourse with no identifiable physical cause. By definition it can only be a problem for bisexual or heterosexual women. Lesbian sexual activity is not defined as 'intercourse'.

Genital pain with sexual stimulation when no cause is found is extremely rare for lesbian women, but it does exist. Women will usually seek medical help. It is important to rule out all the medical conditions referred to above. Rarely, with thorough investigation, it may be found to result from nerve damage due to previous physical trauma or surgery. As with vaginismus, however, the problem may be due to deep-seated fear and past trauma. When meticulous medical investigation has ruled out physical causes, a woman who wants to solve this problem is faced with looking into her past and facing her fears. A competent counsellor or psychotherapist can assist you.

DIFFICULTY WITH ORGASM

In 1977 Sisley and Harris stated '…lesbians always reach orgasm in their love-making'.[17] This is not true! Research indicates that 12 to 16 per cent of women have orgasms rarely or never, whether they are lesbian, bisexual or straight.[18] Eighty per cent of women would like to have orgasms 'more consistently or with more intensity' than they presently do.[19] However, despite this, most lesbian women have a high level of satisfaction with their sex lives.[20]

It is important to realise that for many women, the capacity to have orgasms is learned! Some experience orgasm during their first sexual encounter. Most have to learn about their body. We need to learn what kind of sexual activity we like and what type of partners we are comfortable with. 'Orgasmic capacity in females increases with age.'[21] This is because as women mature they get to know about themselves, their body, their preferences, and how to have an orgasm. Unless there is a relationship problem, a traumatic incident (for example, rape or abuse), or an illness or injury, women who have learned how to have orgasms rarely lose the capacity. Sometimes women find that when they have had a long period of abstinence, it can take them a little while to 'get back into practice'. Often, however, abstinence enhances the intensity of orgasm.

Women experience four common problems with orgasm:

Never coming at all

Anorgasmia is the word that medical practitioners sometimes use to refer to the absence of orgasm. 'Primary anorgasmia' is when a person has never had an orgasm. 'Secondary anorgasmia' is when someone who used to have orgasms no longer does so. Despite the medical progress made in the last century, science is not yet able to explain what causes orgasm to occur. Since we don't really know why it does happen, we do not have precise solutions when it doesn't. There has been little formal research on methods to remedy the absence of orgasm.[22] It is not necessary to know the reason why orgasm is absent in order to change the situation.[23] There are some very effective steps that can be taken.

By far the most common reason for primary anorgasmia is not knowing yourself well enough. This does not necessarily mean sexual inexperience. Even a woman who has 'been around' may not be in touch with her likes and dislikes. She may not know how her body works.

Feeling uncomfortable with sex can cause anorgasmia. There are also a small number of physical, hormonal or developmental problems that may reduce the likelihood of orgasm. These are not common.

If you believe that you have never had an orgasm, first re-read Chapter 6. You may be having mini-orgasms (see pp. 94–95). Even if you are not, don't worry. Before you decide that there is a problem, broaden your sexual repertoire by trying the exercises in Appendix 1.

I would not recommend seeking medical investigation unless you are certain that you've given yourself every chance to relax and learn about your sexual nature. However, if you have frequently been sexually active for several years, are comfortable with yourself and your sexuality and are sure that you have never had an orgasm, consider discussing it with your general practitioner. Unless your GP has an interest in sexual health matters, it may be worthwhile asking for a referral to a sexual health physician who is experienced in problems of sexual function for women. This is a specialised area and unfortunately not all doctors are skilled in it. Seeking out someone who has interest and expertise is worthwhile. Be aware, however, that although some physical causes for the absence of orgasm exist, they are found only rarely.

A number of medications contribute to anorgasmia. Depression (and other mood disorders) may prevent orgasm. Physical illness or impairment may get in the way. There is an association between diabetes and difficulty with orgasm. Alcohol and drug use or abuse is definitely associated with absent orgasm. For most women, however, if a problem exists, it much more commonly has its base in an emotional cause.

Secondary anorgasmia can be due to stress, trauma, relationship difficulties or poor communication. It can also be due to change.

Sometimes when you've been orgasmic with a particular partner in the past, a new partner and different sexual style may lead to difficulties. Humans are creatures of habit and we can become accustomed to doing things one particular way. It can be difficult to tell a new partner exactly what you know will turn you on.

However, sometimes there seems to be no reason that either you, or anyone else, can identify as a reason why orgasm does not occur. Appendix One provides information and suggestions that may assist.

Only coming as a result of specific stimulus

Some women can experience orgasm from a partner's touch, but only from very specific stimulation. Others experience orgasm only from masturbation. For some, orgasm is not possible in the presence of another person, but they can masturbate themselves to climax. Others can experience orgasm with a partner, but only by masturbating themselves.

> **CHRIS:** *I only ever come from clitoral stimulation, and that's when I'm lying on my face and doing it to myself. Gives me the shits. I've never been able to come with a partner. If she can't cop stroking my back while I come, we've had it.*

If you wish, it may be that you can broaden the range of things that give you sexual pleasure through masturbation and sensate focus (see Chapter 6 and Appendix One). If you have never used a vibrator, it is probably worth investing in one. The stronger stimulus will often bring women to climax where other methods fail.

Sometimes the solution is just to accept yourself as you are. With your partner, establish the ways that work best for you to have her involved, and play with those.

Taking a long time to come

This is very common. There is no solution except to allow the time you need. Some women need more than an hour of sexual stimulation before they come to orgasm. If you are a woman whose body will only climax after a lengthy period of arousal, you need to ensure that your partner knows you need a lot of time. We are all different. Some women may have to accept that they will probably never have an orgasmic 'quickie' and enjoy the fact that their sexuality is geared to long, languorous interludes.

Not coming as often as you want to

The majority of women have this complaint. If you want to create change, make sensuality one of the focuses of your life. Everything you do can be sensual. A bath or shower is an opportunity to caress yourself. Dressing in the morning can be your own private celebration of yourself. Undressing at night can be your own private strip tease. Give attention to the sights, smells, textures, tastes and sounds that give you pleasure. On a daily basis, ensure that you do at least one thing for the sensual part of your soul. Doing this reminds you that you are a sensual being. It also makes the pleasure centre in your brain notice that delight can arise from many different stimuli. Extend this adventure of sensuality into your sex life. Be adventurous. Watch erotic television and videos that you might have previously ignored. Be vigilant in your determination to set time aside for self-intimacy. Read the chapter on masturbation. Surf the Internet and see what the sites dedicated to this subject have to offer (see 'Resources'). Let your focus be pleasure, not orgasm.

Other problems associated with orgasm

Headache

There are lots of old jokes about headaches and sex, but it really can be a problem. There is an uncommon condition called 'benign coital headache'. 'Coitus' means sexual intercourse, and in most medical texts, it is defined as penis in vagina sex. This terminology is just evidence of the way in which the medical profession (and our culture) has pretended that lesbians don't exist. Some lesbian women experience this condition. The headache begins very suddenly just before orgasm is about to occur (or sometimes just after climax has taken place). The pain can be very severe and frightening.

> **SIAN:** *I get the most incredible headaches when I orgasm. They are so intense that sometimes I think I am going to die. They really put me off having sex. Eventually I got the courage to tell my doctor about them. She sent me off to see a neurologist who did some tests and then told me what they were. He prescribed some medication to take before I have sex. To my amazement it worked. It was such a relief!*

For some women the headache disappears if she interrupts the sexual activity. Other women find that they are debilitating and may persist for hours afterwards. Some women find that they occur with every orgasm. Others experience them sporadically. If vomiting, drowsiness or dizziness ever accompanies the headache, the woman should see a doctor to exclude more serious problems. However, usually, apart from being painful, the headaches are not associated with serious conditions. There are medications available that may help prevent these headaches.

'Faking it'

> **ANGELA:** *Of course I fake it sometimes! It's just easier.*

Large numbers of women will admit to occasions when they have pretended to have an orgasm. Often the woman just wants to bring a sexual interlude to an end. Women talk of 'faking it' in order not to hurt their partner's feelings or to end a sexual encounter without having to discuss what has happened for them.

'Faking it' is so common that it probably should be included among the range of normal sexual activities. It does, however, raise a number of issues. I think it may be worth considering why a woman chooses to pretend. Does she feel that she needs to appear to be a 'complete sexual being'? I sometimes wonder if a woman who fakes it feels uncomfortable about being herself. If a couple has an agreement to be honest with each other, there is the obvious result that their agreement has been broken.

On the other hand, women say that there is no harm done and it is nobody's business but their own.

Each woman makes her decisions about this within the framework of her own ethics and values.

9

Am I Lesbian? Does it Really Matter?

Am I lesbian?

Many women have no difficulty deciding that they are lesbian. They have always been aware of it. For others, realisation dawns slowly over a period of time as they notice feelings and thoughts arising within themselves. Particular events may precipitate awareness. Meeting a lesbian woman, going to a lesbian social event, and falling in love are all triggers that women have told me about. Each woman reacts differently. Some have no problems at all with the realisation. For others, the new information about themselves can be extremely unsettling and traumatic.

> **JANET:** *I never even thought that I might be lesbian. I was married with kids. I had read about lesbians in women's*

magazines. I had a close friend who I spent a lot of time
with. One day we decided to swap a massage. She kissed me.
I liked it. It went on from there. We were just experimenting.
At the time I thought 'it's not really sex, it just feels good'.
Because it was with a woman I didn't really think I was
cheating on my marriage. Anyway, to cut a long story short,
it blew up in our faces. Eventually my husband found out
(came in and caught us at it). He blew his top, told her
husband. I ended up separating from him. My friend is still
married. My husband used to call me 'slut' and 'dyke'. I
thought, well, if that's what he thinks....I started going to
feminist things like 'Reclaim the night' and met a bunch of
women. I suppose I'm really bisexual, but I really like the
dyke part of me and that's what I'm living now. I've got the
right to call myself lesbian or dyke, whatever I want.

SAM: When I realised what was going on for me I bought
some books and got in touch with a lesbian support group.
Just knowing the other women really helped. There was no
pressure, just women who accepted that they were gay.

KATE: I have an acquaintance who just wants to fuck
around. She lives at home with her husband but really gets
around in the butch lesbian scene. She gets all her connection
and belonging goodies at home. She is really clear that she
doesn't want a relationship. She just wants hot sex. But
women keep falling in love with her.

MARGARET: It (lesbianism) hadn't actually been an option. It
was something I never considered. My husband was like the
old pair of slippers in the corner. There was no passion there,
but the sanctity of marriage and security of my family was
there and I never considered anything else. After I made the
decision to have sex with a woman I guess there was no going
back.

When women are deciding that they may be lesbian, it can be helpful to be aware that there is now quite a lot known about this process. Sexual identity is said to have three elements: gender, orientation and intention.[1]

Gender is the word used to describe how a person sees herself or himself. It depends on the individual's internal psychological experience of being male or female. 'Sex' describes the physical distinction between females and males. It includes matters of anatomy and physiology, for example, having a vagina or penis. People usually become aware of their gender at a very early age. It happens when you think 'I'm a girl' or 'I'm a boy'.

To understand this distinction, imagine a person whose biology is female, but who holds the belief that s/he is male. Which gender would that person experience themselves as? If the person believes he is male and lives in the world as a male, then his gender is male. Physical attributes, social and family factors and the individual's psychological make-up combine to determine the gender that they will experience themselves as.

Part of the task of growing into an adult includes dealing with the following issues: Am I a girl or a boy? Can I accept this label? Do I like this body with its genital parts? How do I feel about the way my family believes that conventional girls and boys should behave? Can I accept the idea that I will grow up to be a man or a woman?[2] Most people answer these questions for themselves without any difficulty. In doing so they establish their core gender identity. This may not be the same as their biological sex.

'Orientation' is a statement about the type of partner that you prefer. If you prefer partners only of the same sex, you are homosexual. If you prefer only partners of the opposite sex, you are heterosexual. However, very early thinkers in relation to sexuality realised it wasn't quite as simple as that. In 1948 Kinsey said that sexuality is a continuum. He suggested a linear scale with seven categories:

- Exclusively heterosexual with no homosexual
- Predominantly heterosexual, only incidentally homosexual

- Predominantly heterosexual, but more than incidentally homosexual
- Equally heterosexual and homosexual
- Predominantly homosexual, but more than incidentally heterosexual
- Predominantly homosexual, only incidentally heterosexual
- Exclusively homosexual.[3]

I believe that Kinsey got it right. However, perhaps it may have been more accurately represented as a bell curve.

The bell curve is used to describe all sorts of normal variation in human, animal and plant biology. It is sometimes called a 'normal distribution curve' and represents the way in which biological variables like height, weight and a large number of other factors are spread in populations.

While I have absolutely no scientific proof, it is my privately held belief that if cultural pressure did not exert its influence, then the way sexual orientation is distributed in our population would be accurately reflected by the bell curve. At one end there would be a small percentage of people who are exclusively heterosexual. At the other end

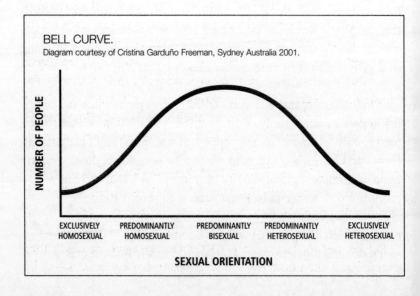

BELL CURVE.
Diagram courtesy of Cristina Garduño Freeman, Sydney Australia 2001.

NUMBER OF PEOPLE

EXCLUSIVELY HOMOSEXUAL · PREDOMINANTLY HOMOSEXUAL · PREDOMINANTLY BISEXUAL · PREDOMINANTLY HETEROSEXUAL · EXCLUSIVELY HETEROSEXUAL

SEXUAL ORIENTATION

there would be a similar percentage that is exclusively homosexual. The rest of us would lie somewhere in the middle. We may have a tendency to be drawn more towards one end or the other. At different times in our lives we may see ourselves differently. We may move around in the area under the curve!

It is not possible to test my theory because cultural influences are a powerful determining factor in the way in which people are prepared to express themselves sexually. Cultural pressure makes it difficult for people to even recognise their own desires. It also determines what people are prepared to say to researchers. It is a powerful force in determining the actions that we will take in our sexual lives.

Intention is a third concept. This takes account of the type of behaviour people want to engage in while having sex.[4] Do you like gentle sexual interaction characterised by the wish to an exchange of enjoyment without pain? Or do you prefer leather, whips, blindfolds and BDSM? Perhaps your taste lies somewhere in between?

Some people will have intentions and behaviours that change little throughout their lives. Others may experiment with, and enjoy, a variety of practices.

Many people reach adulthood knowing their sex (that is, they have physical characteristics such as a vagina or penis) and their gender (they feel like either a woman or a man). They may well be aware of their sexual orientation (the kind of partners that they are attracted to, whether female, male or both). This is not true for all people.

It used to be believed that sex (the physical attributes) were fixed. It was thought that people formed perceptions of their gender by the age of two or three and that this was permanent. It was believed that orientation would be fixed by early adulthood. It was acknowledged that people's erotic intention, and their resulting behaviour, was much more variable.

Things are a lot much more fluid than we thought. In women at least, a significant minority who live their early adult lives in comfortable heterosexuality, discover and delight in a newly found lesbian identity in their twenties, thirties, forties, fifties and sixties.[5]

People may in their adult years decide that a gender which they accepted as a child does not suit their reality. Sex can be changed by gender re-assignment surgery. These things can change back again, (people sometimes have further surgery to reverse an original procedure). Gender and sexuality are new frontiers in science and psychology, and our culture is still coming to grips with the implications of new knowledge in these fields. There are complex issues relating to transgender people, but these are beyond the scope of this book. For more information in relation to transgender issues (see 'Resources'). It is important to realise that in contemporary society, sex, gender and orientation are all very fluid.

Identity formation

Sexual identity formation is the process of deciding whether you are homosexual, heterosexual, bisexual or that you reject labels. It involves determining whether your gender is male, female or transgender. It also involves determining what type of sexual behaviour you like. Lesbian women have a wide variety of experiences.

> **HELEN:** *From the time that I can first remember thinking about it, I always knew I was different. In high school when kids started going out I didn't. I knew I was attracted to girls. I had a miserable time. I just hid it.*

> **SUE:** *When I first thought I might be a dyke, I was really shocked. I found myself attracted to a woman at work. I was 24 at the time. I was really scared. I rejected my feelings; I thought I was sick. That time it was just a crush. Nothing came of it, but the awareness that I could be attracted to women wouldn't go away. I didn't believe that being gay could be okay. I had been brought up a Christian and all the rest of it. It just wasn't part of my world. I became really depressed. I couldn't talk to any of my friends or family about what was going on for me. I talked to my doctor, who only wanted to give me anti-depressants. Eventually, a friend talked me into seeing a counsellor. She was great. It took me*

*a good while to trust her, to actually get the words out of my
mouth that I was attracted to women. One of the best things
was that she wasn't shocked or anything. She seemed to be
quite comfortable with it. She told me about a couple of
lesbian books and magazines, gave me the contact numbers
for a couple of helplines and groups. Basically, she affirmed
that it was an okay option for anyone to choose. She was
realistic; she didn't imply that there were no problems ahead.
But she said that it was one of a range of normal behaviours.*

Vivienne Cass suggests that most people in Western cultures go
through a recognisable process while determining their sexual identity.
She is clear that her views only apply to Western society. Attitudes to
homosexuality vary greatly between cultures. Therefore the way in
which sexual identity forms will also vary from culture to culture.[6]

Before any issue of sexual identity arises, most women assume that
they are one of the majority group, that is, heterosexual.

Dr Cass proposes a theory which sets out stages of sexual
orientation identity formation. Not everyone goes through every stage,
or in the same order. Briefly, the stages that she suggests are:

Identity confusion

The woman starts to notice that there is more than one possibility. It
dawns on her that lesbian and gay people exist. She then begins notice
things about herself and starts to wonder whether she might be lesbian.

Identity comparison

The woman starts to consider the implications of the possibility that
she might be homosexual. She notices that lesbian women and gay men
are a minority group. They are not always welcome in society or treated
fairly. Dr Cass suggests that at this stage, women may experience a
variety of reactions. Some experience 'a sense of comfort as previous
feelings of being different from others become clarified by the new self-
understanding'.[7] Others feel the weight of their estrangement from the
majority in society and experience a sense of rejection, loss and grief.
Some experience fear.

Women have different coping strategies in this stage. Some may accept that they are lesbian, but encourage others to see them as straight. Others say to themselves and others that they are just interested in lesbian sex, but are not really lesbian. Still others tell themselves that they are experiencing a 'one-off' incident that has no bearing on the rest of their lives. (This, of course, may be true.)

> **SALLY:** *I don't think I'm a lesbian. It just so happens that I'm in love with a woman.*

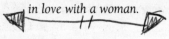

Identity tolerance

At this stage a woman will acknowledge 'I probably am lesbian'.[8] She may not be comfortable with this. Women may begin seeking contact with other lesbian and gay people if this is not already available to them.

> **CATH**: *I can remember travelling on trains in Sydney. By then I knew that I was gay. But I knew hardly any other lesbian women. I was desperate to meet some. I just wanted to know some other women like me. I would sit on the train dyke-spotting. I was never sure. I was never able to catch anyone's eye or start up a conversation.*

Identity acceptance

At this stage the women has an inner sense of self as lesbian. She will often experience fear as she remains aware that she has stepped beyond heterosexuality, where 'power and acceptability lie'.[9] However, she now begins to value her homosexuality, and that of the other people she knows. She often has increasing contact with the lesbian and gay community. She sees other lesbian women getting on with their lives as happy and valued members of both the lesbian and the wider community, and this helps her reach acceptance of her lesbian identity. She may start to tell people about her new view of herself. She begins to experience people relating to her as a lesbian woman.

Identity pride

The woman has accepted herself, but realises that the cultu
her does not. She sometimes becomes angry and frustrated
whole world seems to be straight. She may begin to feel that its 'them
and us'.[10]

The identity that the woman chooses at this stage may be 'lesbian',
'gay', 'dyke', 'queer', 'transgender' or 'bisexual'. She may also choose to
adopt additional labels: 'butch' 'femme', 'vanilla', 'SM', 'top', 'bottom'
and more (see the Glossary). As time goes by, and gender politics
develop, there will be new labels which women may choose to identify
with. Some women reject all labels and simply come to an
understanding that they are not heterosexual in the sense that they had
previously understood.

At this stage homosexual women may fiercely value their lesbian
friends and choose to associate only with them.

> **CATH:** *I went through a stage when I kept my house strictly a
> women only space. I simply would not let men through the
> door. I employed only women tradespeople. I once counted
> how many photos, paintings or drawings of cunts that I had
> on my walls. I had 24, including a nine-foot wall hanging in
> purple and green satin.*

Cass states that at this stage 'the combination of pride and anger is
empowering'.[11] Women often choose to no longer pass as straight. It
often becomes important for them to make public pronouncements of
their lesbian identity by their words, dress or behaviour.

Identity synthesis

As time goes by, an 'out' lesbian woman who experiences positive
reactions from straight people may re-evaluate. The world can no
longer simply be divided into 'good' lesbians, and gay men and 'bad'
heterosexuals'.[12] Those heterosexuals who value her may be included
in her life. Those who do not, receive less of her attention. Her
alienation from those around her may decrease. The level of her anger
may also subside. However, she may have changed her views about the

way society is constructed, and this new view of the world may well continue to inform her decisions and actions. She is aware of oppression and discrimination but now deals with these issues in a less defensive manner. Her need for identification with a lesbian or gay group may or may not reduce. As she walks in the world as an openly lesbian woman, her inner sense of personal identity is strengthened. Cass observes that '…there is a sense of belonging to the world at large and of being more than just a lesbian or gay man. Accounting for self as lesbian or gay is now an integrated part of the whole self and reinforces self-esteem and position in the world.[13]

Integration

Identity = gender, orientation, and behaviour

Not everyone goes through all the stages of identity formation. Women can get stuck at any stage. People have both positive and negative experiences as part of the process. However, when a woman successfully establishes her sexual identity she recognises and becomes comfortable with her gender, her experience of herself as being female (or male). As part of identity formation, she works through to an understanding of which sex(es) she is attracted to (orientation). She works out what kind of sexual behaviour she likes to engage in, and what behaviour is acceptable to her from her partner(s).

Many women feel that they have come to a final resting-place in relation to these issues. Lots of others conclude that there may be continuing change throughout their lives and choose to be comfortable with a fluid sexuality.

A woman who can come to feel at ease with all these internal aspects of herself will have less inner conflict than one who struggles for self-acceptance. She therefore has more resilience to external stressors. She is likely to live her life more successfully, with less tension, and to enjoy her sex life without guilt.

Is lesbianism contagious?

Well, yes and no!

> **CAROL**: *I was on a committee with a number of women. I didn't really consider the fact that they were lesbian. They were just my friends. They were very different to me. They weren't bothered about make-up or fashion so far as I could tell. Only a little interested in clothes. They were interested in the things that they were doing. Feminist politics, a reading group, a music group. They seemed strong, self-confident, self-assured. I respected them. Someone told me that they were lesbian. I didn't really think about what that meant. I became closer to them. I realised that I had a great deal of respect for them. I fell in love with one of the women…*

Some may never think about the possibility of lesbian sex until they meet a lesbian woman. The possibility of a happy, fulfilled lesbian life may not cross the mind of a person who is wrapped up in rural or suburban heterosexuality. However, on meeting someone who acknowledges her lesbian identity, other women, not infrequently, become curious. Some seek to satisfy their curiosity by affairs or relationships. Others ask questions or read about lesbian sex. Some look within themselves. However, unless the capacity for same-sex attraction exists within, it will not be expressed in action.

Among lesbian women there are some firmly held views about affairs and relationships with straight women.

> **LOU:** *I would never have a fling with a straight woman. I'm not there just because they've got interested. They use you; fuck you and dump you. They think you are just there to titillate their curiosity. They don't realise the way in which you can get emotionally involved. They have no idea what being a lesbian is about. Most of my friends feel the same. When I'm thinking about whether I'm interested in a woman,*

part of what I want to know is how long she's been out, and how secure she is in her dyke identity.

JAN: *I really love teaching a new dyke the ropes.*

What's in a name?

There are a number of words that lesbian women use to describe their sexual identity. Common terms in Australia include lesbian, dyke, gay and queer. A term used more recently by researchers is 'WSW' (women who have sex with women). These terms are all defined in the Glossary.

In this book I have tried to concentrate on lesbian sex and to refrain from lesbian political analysis. However, many lesbian women are active in academic and political spheres. Perhaps equal numbers may have no interest in politics and simply live their lives. For political lesbians, openly naming their lesbian identity has important consequences. They stand in the world and declare their sexual orientation. It is believed that every lesbian who is 'out' makes it easier for every other lesbian who follows in her footsteps. It is still an act of courage to name oneself lesbian, dyke, queer or gay. The courage required and costs incurred were much higher in times gone by. This history is intrinsic to attitudes within the lesbian community. Some lesbian women therefore feel passionately about these issues.

In the last twenty years the homosexual community has pushed for an acceptance of diversity. 'Queer' is now a recognised sexual identity. Those who take this name are stating that they are not heterosexual, but declining any further definition.

Many women are comfortable with fluidity in their sexual identity and orientation. Some term themselves bisexual.

There is a polarity of views across the lesbian and gay community about whether the name by which people identify themselves is important.

SYLVANA: *Does identity matter? Depends on who you are, and who you choose to mix with!*

MORGAN: *I think it matters for some people. I think, for me personally no, it doesn't bother me. I wouldn't go out with someone that defined themselves as straight. I think they need to recognise the fact that they are not straight. But other than that, it doesn't bother me and I don't think it is that important. Does the classification make any difference? For some people that's really important. A lot of gay people, especially the lesbian community, won't go out with people that are bisexual.*

CLAIRE: *Yes it matters! I'm old enough now to know what I want in a partner, and in the people that I choose to socialise with. I don't want to waste time with women who are stuffing around. I prefer to mix with women who have some political understanding. I want someone who knows where she is at. I want someone who is not frightened of recognising that she is a dyke. I want someone who is out, and unafraid, and stands on her own two feet in the world!*

LISA: *It's a bit of a joke really. On the one hand, there are the lesbian feminist sex police who say you are only okay if you are a 'right on dyke', and on the other hand, there are the ideologically sound queer police who say that Seventies feminist politics is really old-fashioned and you have to include all diversity. I just ignore the lot of them.*

There is such a diversity of views about whether or not to make declarations concerning sexual identity that the decision rests as a matter of personal choice. Some women feel drawn to declare an identity, and it is right for them to do so. Others live their lives enjoying fluidity of sexual expression and never feel the need to define themselves. I believe that there is no right and wrong in either stance, just a medley of human behaviour that adds spice to our interaction with each other.

10

Coming Out

Coming out is a process. In the lesbian community these words are used to refer to the time when a woman realises that she is lesbian. It also refers to her decisions about sharing this information with others.

Coming out is different for everyone.

MICHELLE: *Well, I was already in a relationship. When I decided to start acknowledging it, my family and lots of my close friends had already guessed. It turned out to be no big deal really.*

SYLVANA: *It was terrible when I broke the news. My stepmother absolutely hit the roof. She called me 'dirty, perverted and disgusting'. She said she wouldn't let the neighbours' children near me. After that first relationship ended, I nearly got married three times. There was so much pressure never to go back into the lesbian world. They said being lesbian did me so much damage and fucked up my life, and everyone else's around me. I ended up having a breakdown.*

MARGARET: *It was really an overnight decision for me. There was no coming out period. That had already been done by other lesbian women everywhere. I didn't have to break the ground. There is already a lesbian community. I don't have to feel any of that shame because other women have already done it. The only thing I had to deal with was how my father reacted. He said, 'I didn't give birth to a man'. At the time I thought, 'Fuck, does he think I strap a dildo on every night?'*

FRAN: *I was about 24 at the time. From things that had been coming up for me, I had pretty much decided that I was probably gay. But I didn't know any other gay women or anything about the scene. I had no idea really. I brought LOTL[1] home to have a look at and my mother found it on my bed. I was outed before I'd even done anything.*

JAY: *Coming out at work was one of the best things I ever did for my career. I'm a middle level manager. When I realised that a few people in my organisation knew, and had been talking about it behind my back, I decided to deal with it head on. I made an appointment to see my most senior boss in his office. I said that I had heard a bit of gossip about me, and I told him I was lesbian and was in a relationship with a woman. Very shortly after that I invited him and his wife over to dinner with my partner and I. We fed them some fantastic food and wine. They really enjoyed the night. After that, there was no problem. I was out. The most senior person in my organisation was okay with it. Nobody could hurt me. I've felt so free ever since. And my career has really taken off.*

MARINA: *I'm an honest person. I want to live with integrity. I couldn't do that before I came out. Not having to lie is so much less stressful than hiding.*

Women who are realising that they are lesbian experience different reactions. Some are deeply troubled by their new knowledge. Some feel scared about what the future might hold. Some women are entirely unworried by it all.

Any major change in one's personal life is stressful. It can be comforting to have someone to talk things through with. You may know someone whose views you value and who you can trust. There are also a number of lesbian and gay telephone counselling services which can help (see p. 239 in 'Resources'). It can be good to talk to women who acknowledge that they are lesbian and who live fulfilled and happy lives. Just knowing how other women have dealt with things can be very useful. There are also a number of organisations that run groups or workshops for women who are coming out (see 'Resources', p. 237 and p. 242).

No matter how you might plan coming out, you cannot predict what it will be like. Every experience is different. People react very unexpectedly. People you think may have difficulty accepting your sexuality will surprise you by having no problems. Others you thought were tolerant will amaze you with their rejection.

Some women feel that their coming out is a lifelong process.[2] First you face yourself. Then bit by bit you tell the truth to others. As long as there are individuals and institutions in our culture that are homophobic, it will be necessary to ask oneself: should I tell this person? Is it worth it? Is it safe?

CLAIRE: *For the most part, I couldn't be bothered hiding. As I've got older I've become a bit stroppier. Usually I feel it's not worth the price that I pay when I'm not out. However, every so often I still find that someone who doesn't know me all that well comes out with a question like 'Haven't you found a good man yet?', or some other personal question. I have to think – now does this person matter enough to me that I will bother saying, 'Well it's not good men that I'm interested in'. Or do I shrug the question off? Even after all these years, I still have to make coming out decisions. And when it's in my professional life, or in my small rural home*

*town, it can still be very scary. It's boring and tedious, and
tiring. But it's still something that I have to face regularly.*

JAY: *There's no way now that I could make any choice other
than to be out. I know what it does to me when I have to
hide. And I know that I'm almost a different sort of human
being when I don't have to. They say that you can't bring all
of yourself to a job when you are not able to be yourself. I
know that's true.*

In years gone by, many lesbians lived their whole lives 'in the closet'.
Lesbian women 'passed' as straight. Coming out, the decision about
who and when to tell was such a big deal that it was the focus of lesbian
poetry, song and many short stories. It's not as hard as it used to be, but
no-one can say it's not stressful. There are some Australian cities and
workplaces where difficulties are uncommon. In some localities,
lesbian and gay people are definitely and visibly ten per cent of the
population. We are respected and accepted for who we are. However,
there are many suburbs, country towns and conservative workplaces
where things are very much more problematic.

Every coming out experience is unique. Each of us has very
different families, workplaces, friends and circumstances to face.
Women may choose to be totally out, not out at all, or something in
between. Many women tell those close to them individually and
gradually. Women choose to come out to some people but not to
others.

FRAN: *I'm not out at work. It's none of their business. People
don't go round saying, 'I'm a heterosexual', or telling me
what they do in bed.*

Fran's point of view is one that lots of gay women hold. It's true, people
don't go around saying 'I'm heterosexual'. They don't have to. It's
assumed. Heterosexuality is the dominant culture. The heterosexual
assumption made by our culture is oppressive. This is sometimes called
'heterosexual privilege'. The result is that LGBT[3] people continually

have to make decisions about whether to correct the wrong assumptions that are constantly made about them. On each occasion, it's necessary to weigh up whether that feels safe.

> **JOANNE:** *Every time I book a motel I say, 'I'd like a double room'. Often when we arrive, they think that there's been a mistake and try and put us into a twin. It happens more in country towns, and overseas in less developed countries. It's a hassle to have to say 'NO, we WANT the double bed'.*

> **VIV:** *It gets boring. Every time a new person asks, 'What does your partner do?' you have to decide on each individual occasion whether you will say 'She's a…'. Or whether you will fudge around it and find a sentence that does not contain a pronoun.*

There are ways. You can ignore the questions for a minute or two and then say 'My partner's a…'. That way you are not using a word that identifies gender. Or you can mumble, so they can't tell whether you've said 'she' or 'he'. Alternatively, you can be so prickly and defensive that no-one ever asks about your private life.

> **JULES:** *I was really scared to come out, but my life changed so much after I did. I realised later that I'd never really been able to be myself at work before. Now I don't have to hide who I am. When everyone else is talking about what they did on the weekend, I can too. Lisa is included in invites to functions and at Christmas time. It's been great. I never realised it would be so easy.*

Reactions of family members and friends vary widely.

The negative reactions

> **LAURA:** *My mother pretended that she hadn't heard what I said.*

It is very common for parents to grieve the loss of your 'normal' life. It sinks in that you may never have the typical white wedding.

> **ROS:** *My father said he hated the thought that he would never, as he imagined, walk down the isle to 'give me away'. My mum cried because she believed I would never have children.*

Some parents feel guilty. They may believe that they have made mistakes or you wouldn't have turned out this way. Others feel puzzled, and have difficulty accepting that they didn't know you well enough to realise that you were gay. Occasionally parents feel hurt and excluded from a major part of your life.

Some families hold the secret of your homosexuality among an inner circle of relatives and will put pressure on a lesbian woman not to disclose to the extended family.

> **ELLIE:** *My family just don't want to hear about it again. I told my mum and dad. They said, 'Okay, you do what you've got to do, but keep it to yourself'.*

It is very, very, common for parents to believe it is just a passing phase. And that you will come through it. It can take many years for parents to let go of these beliefs.

> **LYN:** *Every so often my mum lets it drop that all the people at her church are praying for me.*

Parents and relatives are sometimes angry. Lesbians have been ejected from their homes. Some have been victims of severe violence. Others have written out of a parent's will.

The positive reactions

SUE: *It was a relief. Mum said she always thought I probably was (a lesbian).*

JEMMA: *My mum joined PFLAG [Parents and Friends of Lesbians and Gays].[4] We march together in Mardi Gras. She says she feels glad that I trusted her enough to tell her. It's brought the whole family closer together. We actually have found that we are more real and tell the truth more about hard things than we did before.*

KIM: *A couple of months after I came out to my family, Mum told me about Aunty Prue and Aunty Maisie. They had been 'land girls' in the army and had always lived together after that. Only Prue was really related to us. I hadn't thought about it but Mum said she had wondered if they might be a couple. Mum and I went to visit them. They were in their seventies at the time. As we caught up with each other I let them know about my life, so it was clear to them that I was gay. They never confirmed it one way or another whether they were. But it was one of those really nice family times that you treasure.*

ANNE: *Dad just said he was proud of me that I had the guts to tell them.*

Being out in the workplace

SAM: *I find it's best to be out. Fiona dropped me off at the job interview. When the convenor of the interview panel met me outside the building, I introduced her as my partner.*

SARAH: *In the interview when they asked, 'Have you got any questions?' I asked, 'What policies do you have in place to* *deal with discrimination against lesbians and gay men in the workplace?' I then made it clear that it was a personal concern for me. It was a Christian organisation. I figured it was best to be up-front. I hadn't actually planned on being quite so up-front. I was really surprised when I got the job.*

JAY: *Discrimination? They wouldn't dare. There are laws to protect you from shit like that!*

JENNY: *They made it clear that even when I completed the training course they would never let me qualify. They also made it clear that it was because of my sexuality. I could never have proved it.*

There are a number of things to consider when you are thinking about coming out.

Are you sure of your sexuality or the choices that you've made?
If you are going to come out to people close to you, it may be worth waiting until you know you are probably not going to change your mind. Some feel that there's no point going through all the hassle if you are experimenting.

Do you feel good about your sexuality?
If you feel comfortable about being lesbian, then others will probably be comfortable too. If you feel guilty, angry, defensive or confused, then others are more likely to react negatively. Sometimes it's worth holding off till you are at ease with your sexual orientation. If necessary, seek counselling. There is absolutely no hurry to come out. Take your time.

Why do you want to come out?
People have all sorts of answers to this question. It will probably be helpful for you if you are clear about your motives.

Is it safe to come out?

There are still towns in Australia where lesbians who choose to be out risk being harassed or assaulted. Safety issues may raise themselves in unexpected situations.

> **LISA:** *Friends of mine have just had to move house. It started when they were kissing in their lounge room. They didn't think about it, but they were in front of a large window. The local hoons started chucking rocks on their roof at night and leaving used condoms and horrible letters and things in their mailbox. They decided to move because they didn't see how else they could solve it.*

Safety may not just involve physical safety. Lesbian and gay people still regularly report discrimination in the workplace and in many other situations.

> **MANDY:** *I started coming out at work at the end of my intern year, on the day that they signed the last piece of paper saying I had an unrestricted right to practise medicine. It happened really simply. We were walking out of the hospital. The doctor who was my boss said, 'Is your partner coming to the Christmas party?' I explained that work commitments meant that my partner would not be able to attend. The next question was 'What does he do?'*
>
> *I said 'She's a….'. And that's how I came out at work. Every time someone made the wrong assumption about the gender of my partner I just answered saying 'She…'. Often they actually didn't hear. Usually there was no reaction at all. Sometimes people would go to lengths to tell me that they had friends (or best friends) who were gay.*
>
> *It's significant that I didn't come out till I felt that 'they' couldn't get me any more. When I was a junior doctor, I had sat and listened to a senior colleague talking about how he had discriminated against a lesbian patient. I listened to them make 'poofter' jokes, and talk about other gay work*

*colleagues behind their backs. I was too afraid to challenge
them. I don't know what I would have done if I'd chosen to
do specialty training. I'd really like to think that if I had to
do it again, I'd have more courage.*

*I didn't get through it without confrontation. One day a
work colleague invited me to have a coffee with her. To my
utter astonishment, she then started to explain how amoral
my lifestyle was and the reasons why she felt I should change.*

The possibility that it may be unsafe does not mean you shouldn't be
out. It just means you have to think about what strategies you might
use to cope with the events that could arise.

Do you have any idea what kind of views the person you want to tell holds?

Have you spoken to them about lesbian and gay people generally?

If you are thinking of coming out to someone, it can be useful to
introduce the subject broadly. It may then be possible to gauge their
likely reaction.

Have you thought about what the costs might be?

If you are telling family members, parents or house-sharing people –
are you dependent on them for accommodation or income? Consider
also the possible impact in relation to your employment or education.

Is it your choice to come out?

People will say all sorts of judgmental things like 'You should be honest
about yourself'. Never be pressured by anyone else who thinks you
should be out.

Sometimes people are just curious and are pushing you for their
own selfish, prurient reasons. Ignore them! Only you can know what is
right for you in a particular situation. Sometimes it's simply not safe.
Sometimes the timing is wrong for you. Sometimes you may consider
that the possible costs are just too high for you to accept right now. You
may be feeling too vulnerable to do it now. The reasons don't matter!
The only right time to be out is when you want to be.

During the 1990s, some gay and lesbian organisations went through a period when they coerced their members into being out. Some even 'outed' prominent lesbian and gay figures. This was usually done by informing the media. The theory behind this practice was that the more people who are out, the safer every lesbian and gay person will be. That's probably true. However, most lesbian and gay organisations now agree that only the lesbian woman herself can know, and has the right to choose, when to reveal her sexual orientation. It is not fair, ever, to decide for someone else. You can never know what pressures or particular sanctions the woman may face. No-one else can ever know all the issues that are involved. No-one else has the right to make such an important decision.

Things to remember when you're coming out

If possible, pick your time.
If you are planning to come out to a person who is important to you, it's a good idea to do it when they are not already stressed about some other issue. You will want them to listen to you. They may need time to talk things through with you.

It's not always possible to do this. Coming out often occurs in response to a question or circumstances that you didn't anticipate would arise. It very often takes courage to give an honest answer. And if you don't feel like coming out, it may be appropriate not to answer the question directly. Sometimes women find that their coming out process is a single public declaration:

> **FIONA:** *I came out to my whole university year when we were having a forum on homosexuality. I just couldn't let some of what they were saying go unchallenged.*

Some women feel that coming out is forced upon them:

> **BRIANA:** *My sister walked into the bathroom where I was having a shower and said, 'You'd better tell Mum'.*

I said, 'Tell Mum what?'

'That you're on with Jill and Joanne,' she answered.

'How did you know?'

She said, 'I put two and two together and came up with three'.

There wasn't much I could do. I thought she would tell Mum if I didn't.

So about five minutes later I went into the lounge room and said, 'Mum, there's something I've got to tell you'.

Try to make sure that you have support if it becomes necessary.
Think about who might be there for you to talk with (should the need arise).

Don't come out while either you or the person you are telling is under the influence of alcohol or drugs.
This is not so crucial if the person is only a casual acquaintance. However, if the person is important to you, and you are intending to establish the basis of your future relationship, you both need to be able to think and feel clearly.

Never come out in anger, or to hurt someone, or make them feel guilty.

Consider having some literature or resources available.
If you are coming out to a parent or family member who could have lots of questions, it may be useful to be able to direct them to one of the many pamphlets, books or websites which exist for people who have a friend of relative who is lesbian or gay. It can be easier than doing a lot of talking about it. Many people feel comforted if they are given something to read. See the Resources section.

Let them get to know you first.
If you are coming out to a whole new community, say in a new town or work situation, it is sometimes wise to let them get to know you as

a person first. Once they are able to relate to you as a person, it is more difficult for them to discount you because of your sexuality.

> **PIP:** *When we moved to W… (a rural town, population approx. 3500), we were worried abut how it would go for Melissa (our seven-year-old) at school. Both Carmel and I joined the P&C, and we got on the tuckshop roster and got involved in a few other things at the school. We didn't say much. Just let the other mothers get to know us. If ever the mothers asked us a question we would answer it honestly, but we didn't make a big deal out of anything. After about eighteen months we were really well known in the community and our relationship was accepted. Eight years later we're into all sorts of thing in town. I have to say that we are respected as community members. We haven't really had any trouble at all.*

It's sometimes good to come out to people one at a time, rather than in a big group.
People are often more humane and tolerant when they are by themselves. A large group can sometimes be cruel in its responses.

Don't forget lesbian etiquette.
There is an etiquette in the lesbian community – if you are asked whether one of your friends is gay, give the stock standard answer: 'You'd have to ask her'. Never assume that anyone else is out. Never speak or behave in a way that would out them unless you are absolutely sure that they are always out, in all situations.

11

Making Connections

If you are heterosexual and decide you want a relationship, it's usual to start looking around at people of the opposite sex. You find out who is single. You look for someone with a physical presentation and type of personality that is attractive. When you identify a possible partner, if you have courage, you let them know that you are interested. There is a whole range of verbal and non-verbal strategies for letting people know that you are attracted. I'm not saying that it's easy, but let's face it, if you start chatting to a bloke at a bar, he might not accept your advances, but he probably won't be offended.

It's a bit different if you are lesbian or gay. As well as finding someone who interests you and who is available, you also have to establish whether or not she is lesbian. If not, is she likely to be interested in a same-sex encounter? You have to do some work. You must assess how she is likely to react if you disclose your sexual orientation. Many dykes have stories to tell about being greeted with shock or distaste. Violence is not a common reaction these days but it still occurs.

Throughout recent history, women have used various methods of signalling to each other that they are lesbian. 'Pinky rings', worn on the little finger, were used by women to inform other women of their lesbian status. When in heterosexual company, women would speak about others who were 'friends of Dorothy' or who were 'members of the choir' in order to identify lesbian acquaintances to each other.

More recently, dykes have worn jewellery to identify themselves. Some lesbians wear a 'double women' symbol. Lesbian artists create these in the form of rings, earrings, or pendants. Others wear a labrys. This double-bladed axe was said in lesbian mythology to have been wielded by the ancient Amazon Goddess under her various names.[1] Lesbians have worn it since the 1970s. Some feel that it is a symbol of lesbian separatism. Non-separatist dykes also wear it.

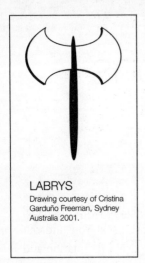

LABRYS
Drawing courtesy of Cristina
Garduño Freeman, Sydney
Australia 2001.

Young dykes tell me that Bonds t-shirts and really short hair are a dress code that may indicate lesbian identity. The trouble is, too many straight women choose the same clothes and haircut.

JANET: *It's not so hard now in the city, there are so many venues and things you can go to.*

SUE: *But a lot of the venues still revolve around alcohol.*

The fact is, you simply can't tell by looking. Some extremely butch-looking women are straight. And some very feminine-looking women are dykes.

LISA: *If I'm interested in someone that I don't know, I usually mention something like Mardi Gras, or some recent article or TV show about lesbians. I watch their body language, and what they say.*

CLEO: *I remember when I was coming out. I was starving hungry for contact with other gay women. Any sort of contact. I would look at women with short haircuts who looked like they might be dykes. I would try to think of ways to start talking with them. I learned, the hard way, that everyone who looks like a dyke most definitely is not!*

ANNE: *There was that old code we used when we were dyke-spotting. You know: DD (definite dykes), PD (Potential Dykes) and BDs (baby dykes, dykes that still have their training wheels on).*

MARY-ANNE: *Yeah, I remember we would sit around talking about who was, and who might be. You laugh about it now, but it was hard feeling like we were such a minority. It was really important to know who else was a dyke too. Gave us a sense of belonging.*

Now that I'm a lesbian, how do I find a lover?

SUE: *What's the problem – just go to Spicy Friday's on a Friday night!*

JEAN: *Not so easy if you don't live in Sydney. When I first looked around T......, it was a desert. I could not identify a single other gay person. It was about three years from when I decided that I was gay to when I felt I had any sort of a dyke social network.*

First of all, it's important to work out what you want. Are you looking for a fast, furious, fun-filled fuck? Or are you seeking a soul mate? Or it may be that you are not looking for a lover at all, but would just like to meet like-minded people. Whichever of these you are after (or even if it is all of the above), the best way is to start mixing with lesbian and gay people. The section titled 'Contacts' in 'Resources' will be helpful.

If you don't already receive the lesbian magazines that are available, see p. 250, also in Resources. Ring up every magazine in your state and subscribe. These publications advertise upcoming events and contact lists for various groups. They are extremely helpful.

Women who live in cities find their social options much broader. It's much easier for urban women to find other lesbians than it is for those who live in rural areas. There's quite a range of clubs in our capital cities now: tennis, ballroom dancing, scuba diving, bushwalking, business dykes, groups relating to various occupations, young lesbians, older lesbians, lesbians with disabilities, spiritual lesbians (Jewish, Buddhist and Christian). Get involved in the lesbian and gay festivals that occur in most capital cities. Don't just go to the events. Volunteer to help.

If you are in the country it may not be so easy. The Resources section will be of some assistance. Other suggestions for rural lesbians include:

- Don't be afraid to go to things by yourself. You have to start somewhere. So get your courage together and go out! People at dances and other events are often very welcoming.
- Realise that in the country you may have to travel. Most regional areas have a gay and lesbian social group. Phone the AIDS Council in the regional centre nearest you. Explain your situation and ask to be given the contact number of the local social group. Then, be prepared to travel to the events that take place in your region.
- Join the lesbian and gay group closest to you. Get involved. Do some of the work. Help to put the newsletter out. Someone who will help fold and stick the stamps on a publication is always valued. Go to every event. Even if it's not the sort of thing that would normally interest you; at least you will meet other lesbian and gay people.
- Offer to help at the local women's dances. Stay and clean up afterwards. You're much more likely to make friends than if all you do is attend the functions.
- Go to a women's music festival. These are advertised in magazines like LOTL (see Resources).
- Go to the Lesfest (on annually), or a lesbian conference.

- Take a trip to the city and go to the large lesbian and gay festivals. Not just the party or parade, but the film festival and cultural events that lead up to the big finale.
- In many towns there is a café, bookshop, pub, gym or other business run by lesbian or gay business people. Hang out there.
- Listen to gay radio (see Resources) – it will tell you what's on.
- The Internet is very, very useful. The Resources section lists a large number of web pages that may be of interest to all sorts of lesbians. You can register on email information lists and newsgroups specifically for lesbians or LGBT people. Once you are on the Internet you can to talk with other people in 'chat rooms'. It's a great way to have contact with other women. Lots of women choose to meet the people that they've been 'chatting' to. If you do decide to meet someone you met on the Internet, use a little caution. Meet in a well-lit public place like a café. Assess how you feel about the person and whether you want to have further contact with them. Don't be afraid to end the association if it's clear to you that you would prefer not to continue it.
- If you live in rural Australia, consider moving to the city, at least until you feel firm and confident in your lesbian identity. You are much more likely to meet lots of lesbians.
- If you are single, consider moving into a shared lesbian household.
- Seek friends, not lovers. Establish a wide lesbian and gay social network. You never know, they may turn into lovers.

> **MEL:** *If you want to make friends, I reckon, don't try and do it at the huge dance parties. They can be a really cliquey scene. I don't actually like it. I find it very unwelcoming and unattractive. It can be really hard to get into those little groups. It can be easier at the smaller dances in the country or in the suburbs. It's certainly much easier at things like the ballroom dancing classes.*

> **ZOE:** *I saw a woman coming out recently. I thought she was great. She was 36, really straight background, all straight*

*friends. I was playing in a band. It was a straight pub. But
we looked really dykey. She came up to us and started
talking. She said, 'So are you all gay ladies?' She didn't say a
lot at first, then she had a few more drinks, and she said, 'I
think I might be bi or a lesbian and I've been broken up with
this guy for a year, and I want to make a move in that
direction'. I just invited her to meet my friends and come out
with us, and away she went. Last I saw her she was most
definitely off and running! She was just really brave. She just
worked it out and just approached us. She seized the
opportunity.*

KAREN: *There are lots of scenes beyond the ones that are
obvious. There are lots of different scenes. The obvious ones
are things like Mardi Gras, lesbian pubs, night spots, some of
the inner city suburbs which have a high dyke population
and so on. But there's a young sporty dyke scene, there's an
older lesbian scene, there's the gay, non-political scene, and
there's the lesbian feminist scene. There's no end to it.*

So what do I do when I find someone?

In the modern world there have been many changes. Nevertheless,
large numbers of heterosexual women wait for men to make the first
move. Many women are too shy to be the one who asks a prospective
partner out, or to initiate intimacy. If lesbian women followed the same
patterns, none of us would ever get it together. Someone has to make
the first move! She may be just as reticent as you are! If you want
anything to happen, you may have to step beyond the behaviour that
is familiar to you, and take some action.

EMMA: *I try to go out as friends first. You have a bit of
leeway. You can work out if you like each other.*

SUE: *I would usually ask her out for coffee. Or a movie maybe. Something casual. Something that you might just ask anyone to. If I wasn't sure whether she was straight or not, I would probably come out to her. I might just mention in passing my ex, and make it clear she was female. And that she is ex. Or I might talk about friends who are a couple and mention both their names. Or some dyke event I've been to recently. Anything to see how she reacts. Usually a dyke will let you know she's a dyke when you do that. Then, if she isn't backing away, I guess you would describe what I do next as flirting. I use my energy to let her know I'm interested in her. I have to detect some interest from her. I absolutely will not go where I am not wanted. But if I get that spark, that awareness that she's interested, then I might push it. If she's responding, at some point I will invade her personal space and touch her. A hand on her shoulder, or arm. Something like that. See how she reacts. Take it from there…*

CLAIRE: *I don't have any problems. If I meet someone I want to know better I will just ring them and ask them out to dinner. It felt very strange the first time I did it. I was obviously asking her out on a date. I think both she and I were surprised that I was doing it. But she accepted and we went out. I really enjoyed it. So did she. But we obviously weren't suited to each other at all. Still, it cut through a lot of crap. I've been doing it that way ever since.*

There are many different ways to initiate closeness. Making the first move always carries with it the risk of rejection, so it's best to act when you are feeling emotionally resilient. As time goes by, and experience is gained, lesbian women often find their own individual style. It is a matter of experimenting to find out what you are comfortable with.

12

Young Lesbians

Sometimes young lesbians or bisexual women worry that they are the only ones in the universe who feel the way they do.[1] Don't worry – **you are not alone**! Being sexual is normal. Being same-sex attracted is normal and okay! But it can be hard in a world where people tell us that the only 'proper' sexuality is heterosexual. The challenge is to connect with others who are same-sex attracted. There are lots of other lesbians out there. You can find contacts, websites and publications for young people on p. 261.

Six vibrant young women have, with their contributions, helped me write this chapter. Hannah: (17), Helen (16), Jules (21), Lisa (22), Melissa (25) and Morgan (17).

Women and girls start to consider that they might be lesbian at different ages. Many young women speak of being surprised when they notice their own interest and sexual feelings towards women.

> **MELISSA:** *At school, I didn't even know that lesbians existed. I didn't know women could love women. I remember when I first had my licence, driving along the road, and my head turning to notice a woman running. And I started questioning why my head would turn at a woman. And then*

I went to a function and I got that whole little butterfly belly thing, that whole 'Oh my god, I'm really turned on by this woman'. So I guess that made me start thinking about it. That was when I was about seventeen.

Other young women have always known that they were 'different'. Their sexuality has always been directed towards women and hasn't been much of an issue for them.

HELEN: *I've always seen myself as a tomboy. I've never really fitted in with most of the girls. When they started those personal development classes at school I knew most of the hetero stuff didn't apply to me. I just wasn't pulled that way. Ever.*

MORGAN: *Well, I never really made a conscious decision. It had always been an option. I never had to think, well, I could be straight, I could be gay, I could be bisexual. it was just always there. So I guess I just experimented. In Year 9 when I moved to Sydney, there were gay people at school and I became close friends with some of them. And with one girl I started having, not a relationship, but something. I don't know what you'd call it. A sexual romance, but not serious. So I guess I just kind of experienced stuff first, before I really considered what ramifications that might have.*

It can be really hard to contemplate sexuality that is different from the norm. Everyone knows that adolescence is a stressful time. There is the stress of school – exams and employment choices may be life-shaping. You are working out what sort of a person you are, in all sorts of different ways. Relationships with parents and carers are not always easy. So young women who find themselves attracted to other women may feel shaken to the core. A discovery that your sexuality may be bi, lesbian or queer can meet with disapproval. The stress can feel too much.

MELISSA: *I had a friend who just sat down with me. She was sitting there saying, 'Oh if I woke up and thought I was a lesbian, it wouldn't bother me', and I was just sitting there thinking, 'Well fuck, it bothers me! It bothers me!'.*

LISA: *I just couldn't cope. I had no idea that there was anyone I could have turned to. There was no-one I knew I could talk to. My whole future seemed completely black. I just couldn't see any point in going on. I took an overdose and ended up on life-support in intensive care for days. It all ended up with them knowing why because the psychiatrist got it out of me – that it was because I'm gay.*

Sometimes young women who are attracted to women feel very down and depressed. This can be because it seems that no-one understands. It can be from feeling so alone. It can be because of fear of the reactions of family, friends and society.

Feeling suicidal is common. **If you are feeling so low that you are considering harming yourself, reach out – there are people to talk to!**

LISA: *I'm so incredibly glad that my sister found me in time. I was unconscious. They told me I was almost dead. When I woke up I knew somehow, like really from the bottom of my soul, that it was not worth killing myself for. I would never take another overdose. I came through the whole thing. And while it was shit for a while, my family survived.*

Many of the help lines have 1800 numbers, which are free to call. The number does not appear on your parents' phone bill. If you feel you can't ring from home, use a public telephone booth. Some services have numbers starting with '13.' The cost of these calls is only for a local call, no matter where you are calling from. However, numbers starting with 13 **will** appear on the phone bill.

Most states have a Gay and Lesbian Counselling Service (see the Resources section). Lesbian women and gay men staff these services.

Reach out, there are people to talk to. Even if times are tough, there are people who can help. Here are some of those that young people talk to when things get tough.

RING:
KIDS HELP LINE ON 1800 55 1800,
OR LIFELINE ON 131114.

Both are open seven days a week, 24 hours a day.
There are services especially set up for young lesbian and gay people. Check these out in the Resources section at the back of this book.

Gay and lesbian counselling services are usually staffed by volunteers, so the phone lines are usually open for limited hours only. Making a call can be a good way of getting to talk to someone like you. Lots of young people say that talking to another lesbian or gay person has been really, really important to them.

Knowing that lots of other women have found their way through the same problems helps. Learning the solutions that other women have used helps. Just having the chance to speak to someone about it helps.

Another thing that helps is information! Look on p. 261 to find resources for young people. Get on the Internet and find some of the fantastic websites created by and for young lesbian and gay people.

Even when it seems that there is nowhere to turn there are options:

JULES: *There was definitely no way I could talk to anyone at home. I was totally isolated. Then I worked out that I could go downtown to the one and only Internet café and get on the Net. I was safe from my parents springing me. It saved my sanity, gave me something to hang onto, until I finally left home.*

Everyone feels down when things are really hard. It's normal! However, sometimes things can be really tough. It's important to recognise when it's time to take action! Look at the list below:

- Has the feeling of sadness or being down been present continually for more than a few weeks? Is it accompanied by feeling hopeless or worthless?
- Do you feel you have no energy and no interest in your usual activities?
- Are you having difficulty sleeping? Or do you find that you are sleeping all the time?
- Have you noticed that you don't feel like eating at all and are losing weight that you didn't intend to? Or have you been eating recklessly and gaining large amounts of weight?
- Have you felt as if you might harm yourself?

If you said 'yes' to three or more of the questions, then it's time to **reach out to the people trained to help. Talk to someone you trust about how you are feeling.** Ring one of the help lines on the previous page, or in the Resources section.

Other options that you might choose to consider are youth workers, school counsellors, health workers at your women's health centre, or workers at community health centres or neighbourhood centres. Some (but not all) local doctors can be really supportive and helpful.

It is important to talk to someone who feels safe to you! People trained to help can recommend ways to start changing the situation.

Young city lesbians may have very different experiences from women in rural areas. In the country, lesbian or gay people in the community may not be as visible. With very few role models, and no-one that you know who is lesbian or gay to talk to, you may feel alone. In rural areas, young women may decide that they can't discuss their sexuality with the local school counsellor or youth workers. Sometimes young women who live in country towns fear that their confidentiality may not be respected. This fear may be well founded – trust your instinct on this. **But don't despair!** Whether you live in the country or the city there is someone you can talk to. There are contacts listed on p. 237. Also read Chapter 11, 'Making a Connection'.

Young people in rural areas connect with the vibrant lesbian and gay community through the web. If you surf the Net you will find many sites. For a start, see p. 250 (Internet sites).

Sometimes young women who wonder if they might be lesbian feel a great deal of fear. They may experience a strong need to be secretive about it. This gut reaction may be recognition of the fact that it is simply not safe for you to tell people about your feelings right now. A major difference between lesbian young women and lesbian adults is that young people may still be dependent on others for their housing, education and financial support. If you feel the need to keep it a secret, that's fine. Read Chapter 10, 'Coming Out'. Take your time. There is no reason to take any action until you are ready and feel sure about it. The time will come when you know what you want and feel it is safe to take action.

In fact, it is very likely that you don't have to decide right now. Many young people feel sexual attraction to people of the same sex, but this doesn't necessarily mean they are lesbian. Some young women are absolutely sure, having always known that they are attracted to women. Others are not so sure. Feeling attracted to women does not make you a lesbian. Having sex with women doesn't make you a lesbian. Feeling attracted to men does not make you heterosexual. You don't have to make a decision or accept a label. It is okay to explore your sexuality for as long as you like.

It's also worth remembering that sexuality is fluid. It may be that you go through a period of relating to people of the same sex and then decide that you prefer relating to men. The opposite can occur. You may conclude that you are really bisexual. You may never in your life reach a final decision. That's all okay. There is no reason why you have to reach a conclusion.

Among some people in our culture, particularly young people, there is now an attitude of flexibility in relation to their sexuality.

JULES: *There's this whole thing now at uni of sleeping with women. Half the girls are bonking with each other. And you* *can see that some of them are looking round and working out whether or not they are lesbian or bi. And lots are not.*

Many young people refuse to accept stereotypes.

> **HANNAH:** *I don't really like to use labels - I will not let anyone stick one on me. I would say, really, if I said anything at all, that I'm just a sexual being, and even that is too much of a label...*

> **MELISSA:** *...and having really long curly red hair I wasn't seen as a dyke, of course. And eventually I moved to Sydney because being in P......, it wasn't safe to walk down the street holding hands. My partner was not what you consider a typical dyke-looking woman either. I found Sydney really, really hard because I'd go to a club or somewhere and they'd say, 'You do realise this is a lesbian venue?'. And I'd think, 'yes I do! What the fuck am I supposed to do to walk in here? Do I have to have "lesbian" tattooed on my head?'*

While some women reject labels and stereotypes, for others it is very important to decide to identify themselves as lesbian, dyke or gay.[2] There are many reasons for this.

> **HELEN:** *I do see myself as lesbian. I identify as a dyke. I have made decisions about it and I want to be out and proud. For some people it is about belonging, identifying with the gay community. But it's not that for me. It's just that I want to say loudly and clearly to the world: 'This is who I am'.*

> **JULES:** *My relationship with Lisa is one of the most valuable things in my life. I don't want to hide something that is so important to me. So I eventually decided that the only way was to be out as a dyke.*

You may be thinking about the issues of identity and coming out. They are discussed further in chapters 9 and 10. Some women find that they worry about the issue of identity until they reach a firm conclusion. Others don't care. They just live their lives and work it out as they go. Just use the approach that feels right for you.

There are a number of matters that young women have to confront that differ from those faced by older lesbians, which I'll now talk about in more detail.

Parents

It's difficult to know how parents will react to learning that their daughter identifies as lesbian. They may react with shock, grief, anger or disbelief. They may have already guessed. They may feel guilty. They may be asking what they did wrong. They may worry that you will never have a 'proper' marriage. They may fear that you will never give them grandchildren. They may be afraid for you. Some women are surprised how accepting their parents are. Some mothers are lesbians themselves (or may wish they had the courage to be).

You may have some idea of what their reaction will be from the things that they've said about lesbian and gay people in the past. You may think they are quite open-minded about same-sex relationships, but don't be surprised if they react differently when it is you! However, they may cope better than you could ever have imagined – it may be no problem for them. Or they may not take it very well at all.

> **JULES:** *All I can say is don't underestimate them. My parents are really conservative. I told them about Lisa because I couldn't stand the lying. My father said never to come under his roof again if I was still living a corrupt lifestyle. So for about two years I never went home. Then, at my brother's wedding, Lisa and I started talking with my mother. Later that day, my father said they both had been feeling that they'd done the wrong thing by me. They invited us for dinner. We've been rebuilding a relationship for the*

> *last nine months. It's been slow. I won't say there's been no*
> *damage, but what is happening now is fantastic.*

PFLAG (Parents and Friends of Lesbians and Gays) was established by
parents who want to support their lesbian and gay children. The
Resources section of this book contains information for parents.

When parents have issues with lesbian and gay sexuality, remember
that it is really their issue, not yours. You don't have to fix it for them.
You don't have to change who you are to suit them. You don't have to
be a counsellor for your parents. It is up to parents to do their own
work to educate themselves. It is up to parents to look at themselves.
There is a certain level of tolerance that is expected in our culture now!

> **MELISSA:** *I ended up saying, 'I accept myself. I love you. Get*
> *beyond it. Come back to unconditional!'.*

However, it may be wise to give them time and keep a compassionate
door open:

> **HANNAH:** *It helped that my sister came out as a dyke about*
> *nine years ago. She never stops talking with my parents*
> *about it. Giving them books. Sending them to movies. They*
> *were total dinosaurs at first, but they are coming along.*

Friends

For young people, having a group of friends is very important. What
your friends think about you can seem crucial. As you decide who you
are, you may realise your values are not the same as those of your
friends. Parts of the dominant culture are still disapproving of lesbians.
If your friends hold intolerant views, you may have to decide whether
you want to hide your lesbian identity or find a new group of friends
who will accept you for who you are.

MELISSA: *I had friends that I thought, from things they said, would be intolerant. It ended up that they were pissed off at me when I did tell them, for not being out before. Some friends love you for who you are. Most don't run away, though a couple did.*

School, TAFE, university and work

Schools are institutions. They usually don't encourage diversity. Traditionally, students wear uniforms. Individuality of dress is suppressed. The function of schools is to teach not only information, but also the morals and values of the dominant culture. In some schools, people who are different find that they have a very difficult time. If a same-sex attracted young person experiences abuse or harassment, there is a seventy per cent chance it will be at school.[3] Girls are less likely to be abused than boys (fifty-three per cent versus eighty-one per cent).[4]

Morgan has just completed her HSC. She moved from a school in a large town outside Sydney to a city girls high school. She speaks about the schools she attended:

> *At O…….. they like to classify you. You are gay or you are straight. They are quick to judge and they are very, very bitchy about it. If you are gay at O……., and you come out, or somebody knows, everybody will know. And they won't treat you the same, you know; a lot of people that you thought were your friends won't be your friends any more.*
>
> *Whereas in Sydney you say you are gay and you might lose one friend. But you are not going to lose a lot of your friends. If a girl was going out with a girl, or a girl was going out with a guy, it didn't make any difference, not to the majority of the year. There were a few people who would have their little bitch about it, but everybody else was fine.*

> *In Sydney, you know, it depends what school you go to.*
> *You might have trouble at some of the private schools or*
> *Catholic schools.*
>
> *At O........ I had such shit – like being left out of sitting*
> *at tables, or being ignored, or being bitched at, or being*
> *teased, you know that kind of thing. Generally, I didn't sit*
> *with people in my own year. I sat with people a couple of*
> *years above, who were not, you know, the popular ones in*
> *their year. It wasn't exactly a friendly environment. That was*
> *a really difficult time, because at the end of the day, everyone*
> *wants to be at least accepted.*

Reactions at TAFE and university may depend on where the institution is located. In many cities, there are active lesbian and gay student organisations at tertiary institutions.

Both older and younger lesbians have to deal with reactions in their workplaces. Young women often have less power and seniority. They are more likely to be in positions where they feel they have to continually prove that they are good enough to keep the job. They may be apprentices, trainees or students. All these positions rely on the good opinion of others. Sometimes it is necessary to make careful decisions about who you tell.

> **MORGAN:** *I worked in a fish and chip shop with a bunch of*
> *straight Aussie guys and a few surfie girls. They were really*
> *homophobic. On one of my early shifts, I mentioned I was*
> *going to go to Mardi Gras, and they said 'Why are you going*
> *to Mardi Gras, are you fucking gay or something?'. So I*
> *decided not to tell them. I invented a boyfriend called Adam*
> *for a long time (who was Amy). They had issues with all gay*
> *people. If a male walked in the shop who looked slightly gay,*
> *they would start calling out 'gaylord' and all that shit, and*
> *would tease them. It was a really unfriendly environment to*
> *work in. And I think they might have found out that I was*
> *gay because they stopped giving me shifts. Became really*
> *rude to me whenever I went in. Just that kind of thing. Not*

so much out and out, 'Oh you are fucking gay', just being really rude about everything. I left. Now I'm working in a fantastic job. It actually markets to the gay community. It's great to work in a place where it's not an issue.

Drugs and alcohol

Recent studies in Australia and the United States indicate that same-sex attracted young people are more likely to use drugs and alcohol than those of the same age in the general population.[5]

> **HANNAH:** *I end up taking eccy,[6] or smoking yarni[7] when everyone else is.*

> **JUDE:** *I used to use a fair bit of e. The party atmosphere can push you into it. Your friends can push you into it. These days I make my choices about what I'm going to take and what I am going to do. I reckon that if you are going to do it, don't do it in an already fucked-up state. If you are feeling low, the after-effects of chemicals can make you much worse. Eccy Tuesday[8] can be a pure bitch. If you are going to party and live in Sydney, check out the Sydney Star Observer and the other gay press. They will often mention if there is crap around.*

It is up to you if you use alcohol, tobacco or illegal drugs. You have a choice. If you do choose to use illegally made or grown drugs, remember, they are not predictable in their effects. Be well informed and know the risks. Have a couple of safety rules. Make sure that someone you trust is with you. Start with a little bit first, so you can gauge how strong the effect is.

If you think alcohol ar other drugs are getting in the way of you living life the way you would like to, phone the free, confidential 24-hour Alcohol and Drug Information Service on 1800 422 599.

Jokes, harassment, vilification, violence

People sometimes make derogatory jokes about lesbians and gay men. It can feel as if they are talking about you. This could be true, or they could be talking about someone else. In Australia in 1998, almost half (forty-six per cent) of the same-sex attracted young people interviewed by Lynne Hillier said that they had been verbally abused.

Harassment is behaviour that offends, humiliates or intimidates you because of your sexual identity. Vilification is a public action that is likely to cause hatred, contempt or ridicule towards you or other lesbian and gay people because of your homosexuality. Both are against the law (see Resources, p. 242). You have the right not to be physically abused. The law exists to protect you.

No-one can tell you how to respond to harassment or vilification, but there are several important things to remember. First, ensure your physical safety. Verbal abuse may sometimes occur just before the perpetrator starts to become violent. Be alert to the possibility that verbal harassment can escalate to physical violence. If your instinct says 'get out of here', trust it. Whatever it takes, remove yourself from the situation. Later, think about it, and decide if you want to assert your rights. Information that will help is on p. 260. Visit the Anti-Violence Project website. It has good information about harassment and violence, and excellent suggestions about what to do.

It is very 'street-wise' to notice people's body language. Be aware of your surroundings. You may be able prevent or defuse violence before it occurs. If you feel that there is a possibility someone could be violent, projecting self-assurance and confidence can sometimes help to get you our of a sticky situation. However, trust your instincts; sometimes simply backing off or running away is safest.

In Hillier's study, thirteen per cent of participants said that they had been physically abused.[9] This can occur at school, on the street, and at social events.[10] Less than half (forty-four per cent) of the perpetrators were strangers. In ten per cent of instances, young people reported that the physical abuse had occurred at home and family members were the perpetrators. These statistics mean that violence and abuse are a significant risk for young lesbians. So always be ready to take steps to ensure your personal safety.

Self-esteem

Young women often have difficulty attaining healthy self-esteem. Part of the task of becoming adult is to work out how your individual values differ from those of parents and families. Young people look around at the world, and the people they know. They then decide what is important to them and how they want to develop. The media portrays the ideal young female as slim, fit, employed in a great job, athletic, attached to a fantastic boyfriend...and on it goes. Our culture's standards for what it takes to be socially sought after are just too high for most people to meet. Sometimes, young women feel that a lesbian sexual preference may damage their positive self-image. If you feel that your self-esteem has been diminished because of your sexual identity, it may be worth remembering that it's not you that has the problem – it's society that is deficient and intolerant. On p. 257 (in 'Resources') there are publications listed that provide helpful tips to bolster your self-esteem.

When you are young, and coming to terms with a lesbian sexual identity, the future can seem daunting. But there is a way through. Huge numbers of lesbian women and gay men have lived through the hard times of deciding how to deal with these issues. Many of us live life vibrantly and successfully. So can you.

13

Older Lesbians

I n writing this chapter I have been privileged to hear the stories and wisdom of a number of remarkable women. Some were leaders of lesbians. Others quietly worked, raised their children, ran their homes and lived their lives. Bev (58), Claire (62), Marian (65), Louise (76) and Sylvana (53), have given me their perspectives. Like other older women, senior lesbians endure our culture's attitudes towards ageing. Some feel that there are special differences, which arise from their lesbian life story. Others have told me that as time goes by, the differences have felt less important to them.

AGEING

CLAIRE: *I was lucky. As a young woman I had some magnificent older women role models. I used to have a photo of Jan standing on the mountain, just wearing shorts and swinging an axe with the light of the setting sun on her grey hair. She taught me about women's strength. She taught me that we can get things done. I always used to fall for older* *women. Short, steely grey hair was one of those things that has always attracted me in a woman. There was a time when I regularly fell in love with older women. So as I started to age it held no terrors for me. I didn't see myself as less sexually desirable, because ageing women had always turned me on. I didn't see myself as less powerful, because ageing women had been my mentors.*

In Western society, ageing is usually viewed in a negative manner. It is portrayed as a process of physical and intellectual decay. Such a perspective admits only one facet of the many that could be noted. It does not see the wisdom. It neglects the richness of experience the passing years may bring. It ignores the joy and light-heartedness that some feel when letting go of 'do-ing' and busy-ness. It ignores the experience of completeness that some enjoy in letting go of life itself.

Older lesbians and other older women are challenging society's rigid stereotypes about ageing. Older lesbian women may be working less, perhaps going out less, and living more quietly than in earlier years. However, many have full days and lives busy with the things that they want to do.

'Ageism' is the process of discriminating against people because of their age, or the fact that their physical appearance is aged.

LOUISE: *I'm doubly invisible now. For so many years, my lesbian identity, the quintessential part of my core, was not visible to the world. Now as a 'little old lady' I am almost unnoticed. Amazing how I can wait for service, say in a shop, and an 18-year-old boy will walk up and be served first. It's as if they just don't see me. Interestingly, I don't have a problem with it if Maree and I are riding the Harley.*

Ageism is a product of our culture's myth that physical beauty is a commodity that belongs only to the young and slim. It is also to some extent a product of our society's preoccupation with profit. Many categorise people by their status; one way in which we determine this is by occupation. Frequently, when meeting new people, our first question is 'What do you do?' In the dominant culture, people who do not contribute to the paid workforce are often not valued. Older lesbian women may define their value and contributions differently. Some will respond to such questions by telling of their daily lives, and making it clear that as far as they are concerned, their activities are equal in value to paid work.

Throughout their lives, many women and men, lesbian, gay and straight, attempt to control what happens to them. Some want to prevent themselves being harmed by life's fluctuating fortunes by, for example, accumulating assets: houses (to be safe from the whims of landlords), cars (to control how and when they travel), health insurance (to have a choice of professional carer). The list goes on and on. But lesbian women may often have made different choices from those who live in the mainstream community. Some have elected to share in co-operative lands or housing rather than to buy houses. Some have chosen to do political, healing or community work rather than to accumulate assets.

As the physical body ages, the capacity to remain in control of life's events may diminish, and sometimes evaporate. Some women don't try to control. They flow with life's changes. They adapt! They create! They invent!

> **CLAIRE:** *If I have any wisdom at all, if I've gained any awareness at all out of all of my life's experience, then it's that I've learned to accept the natural order of things. I try to look at what is in front of me, and accept it without wanting it to be anything other than it is.*

Our culture fears ageing, and the letting go that it implies. Some therefore find it easier to distance themselves from those who are ageing. One way of doing this is to see aged people as stereotypes. Once a woman's physical appearance takes on certain characteristics, it is easier for those who fear the ageing process to see her as inconsequential. This way, it is not necessary to relate to her, and to acknowledge her wishes, needs, wants and fears.

Many lesbians have had to surmount the barriers of the stereotypes imposed on them because they are women. They will often have also been victims of prejudice because they are lesbians. They therefore readily recognise the process of discrimination that occurs as a result of their status as ageing women.

> **LOUISE:** *It's just another one of those things where I think that society can go and get stuffed.*

Contrary to the stereotypes, most ageing people do stay in their own homes (ninety-three per cent).[1] The vast majority (ninety-seven per cent) participate in community activities.[2] More than half of all ageing people in Australia require no assistance of any type. If an aged woman does require assistance with some of her activities, it is most likely that it will not be in relation to personal care.[3] More usually, it will be a need for assistance with property maintenance or transport.[4] We are not as vulnerable as the urban myths would lead us to believe: women over the age of fifty-five are the least likely of any group in our culture to be the victim of personal crime.[5]

Christianne Northrup writes about cultures that value postmenopausal women.[6] Referring to Celtic culture, she notes that

> *...the role of the postmenopausal woman is to go forth and re-seed the community with her concentrated kernel of truth and wisdom.*[7]

She also states:

> *In some native cultures, menopausal women were felt to retain their 'wise blood,' rather than to shed it cyclically, and were therefore considered more powerful than menstruating women. A woman could not be shaman until she was past menopause...*[8]

In some tribal cultures, menopausal women were the matriarchs who audited the tribe's choices. They were not afraid to stand against decisions that they felt 'did not serve life'.[9] They accepted responsibility for teaching younger women the paths of truth and spirituality.

Everyday issues

Older lesbians often say that they find it difficult to meet other older lesbians. The bars and venues advertised in the lesbian and gay press may not be attractive to them.

> **CLAIRE:** *I don't really like venues that are loud and smoky. I don't really relate to the music. You do get some older women there, but there are overwhelming younger women. And you know, I don't really think that the young city dykes are that comfortable with us older dykes either.*

Often, older lesbians have well-established networks of friends and socialise within them. However, unpredictable events can disrupt comfortable routines: relationship break-up, moving to a new town, or the end of a long and intense period of work or study. Sometimes older women are just finding their lesbian identity. All of these events can mean it's necessary to seek new connections. It can be hard to find the older dykes community (p. 253 gives useful suggestions).

> **LOUISE:** *My previous relationship lasted for eighteen years. We had a group of friends that we mixed with. When the relationship ended it was too painful for me to keep seeing the friends we had both been close to. I kept in touch with them, of course, but I needed to meet new women. It took me more than two years to finally shake myself back together. Then I went to ballroom dancing classes for dykes and to the bushwalking group. I also went to a couple of conferences. Before long I was back into it.*

Like heterosexual women, older lesbian women are concerned about finances and housing.[10]

CLAIRE: *I really do worry about the future sometimes. Because I have made the choice to be a dyke, I have no children. I have chosen to be single for some years now. I don't want to end up as an old lady, unable to look after myself, in a hostel or nursing home with all heterosexual people. The fact is, they cannot understand my life. My history and life story have been so different from theirs. I really want to organise it so that there are some dykes around me at the end of my days.*

MARIAN: *We were concerned about older women's housing. We were looking at creating the old dykes' home. But when we did our own survey of the older dykes we knew, we found we were a small group with very diverse needs. The variety of things that people wanted was too large. So some of us have just all booked into the same establishment. It was the quickest way.*

SYLVANA: *I was a freelance photographer for women's groups and environmental groups. I committed a lot of my life to it. Sometimes I got paid. More often than not I wouldn't. I spent ten years dedicating my life to the women's movement. Hence I now do not own my own home. I do not have the financial backup of fifteen years of a wage, plus the super that goes with it. The most important part of my life, in which I had so much energy, was spent on it. I've come out of it socially satisfied but financially impoverished. I've got heaps and heaps of experience, but not the assets that some of my friends have accumulated by being into law, medicine or other areas where they worked for heterosexual society.*

Some lesbian women will choose to be single. This may have its own special challenges.

CLAIRE: *I feel that I may well not choose to have another relationship. I can't imagine myself having a live-in* *relationship. Part of my thinking is that in many tribes, a sixty-two-year-old woman is aged, almost dying. It's an age that you might get left out in the snow, or be left as they walk on. In other cultures you would be seen as a matriarch, a source of wisdom. I don't think I fit the bill in our culture. But I accept that it's okay to come to a point where you may choose a path of not relating. And it can be a conscious choice. It may be about what you get, by not relating, in terms of wisdom. You can't turn inward, to really sit with your own self, if you are connecting with someone else all the time. I have a few friends who are single. I've been talking and thinking about these ideas for a while. It's against the mainstream though. People don't understand why you would choose to be alone if you had an option. And it has its problems, one of which is that you are more vulnerable.*

Changing

Ageing is a process of change. It affects women's lives in a large number of ways. It does have an impact on the way women interact sexually. Mainstream medical authorities state:

Orgasmic capacity in females increases with age.[11]

The nature of orgasm may change.

MARIAN: *Orgasm has changed for me. It feels different. Mellower. Longer lasting.*

For both lesbian and heterosexual women, the frequency of sexual activity diminishes with age.[12]

MARIAN: *I'm a bit of a sex maniac. And I'm well known for it. My friends think of me as someone who is very, very oriented towards sex. I was a late starter. I came out when I* *was forty. So I had close encounters with a lot of women in a short time. Until I hit menopause, I was usually the initiator. I didn't take HRT and my sex drive really dropped off. I would be walking down the street and I didn't feel it like I used to. The fire in the belly (a bit further down really) wasn't there. I sort of soldiered on with the whole thing. Then about five yeas ago I met my present partner. We both found the same thing. It's a matter of energy. I'm sixty-five and she's fifty-eight. We were just so tired with working full-time, kids, friends…I became really aware that sex after a hard day's work wasn't going to be too good. Then I got a medical condition. I was advised by the specialist to go on HRT. For the last two years, it has absolutely put my sex drive back where it was. But still, quite honestly, if we manage to get it together once a month we're doing well. When we do it though, we do it really well. In between we do a lot of cuddling.*

BEV: *When I first came out, my lesbianism was central to my life. It was a demonstration of my absolute unwillingness to subject myself to men. Now my whole approach is different. Sex and sexuality is quite peripheral in my life.*

One of the most visible things are the physical changes.

CLAIRE: *Your skin changes you know. And you stiffen up. But you adapt.*

Ageing often has an effect on our politics:

MARIAN: *I feel a bit burnt out. I'm still always involved in at least one lesbian feminist organisation. A lot of us old activist types just feel like getting on with our lives now. I finally realised it's okay to spend time for myself. Women sometimes have a lot of trouble realising that.*

BEV: *In Brisbane I had been a crew-cutted, blue singletted, 'look at my tits and I'll punch you' dyke. I'm less adversarial now. I can accept that people are all making their way the best they can, even if I disagree strongly with what they do. And these days my inner process ranks alongside my commitment to social justice.*

Women have told me that the things that are most important to them in life have changed.

SYLVANA: *A successful relationship. I don't want the highs and the lows and that sort of enormous stuff that comes with lesbian drama, because I'm worn out, I'm tired, and emotionally I don't want to go through that panic. By successful I mean something that I can live with long term, and plan a future, and be happy with and satisfied. And realise that the grass isn't always greener and that you can actually have a love, and a certain amount of harmony and unity. And you can enjoy it, expand on it and build things together. And that the relationship that you've got together is growing, and that the trust that you've got between each other is getting deeper, that you're happier as time goes on.*

BEV: *The absolute driving force of my life used to be social justice, in particular anti-racism, feminism and lesbian liberation. I wanted to put all the wrongs of the world to right in my lifetime. Now I find myself focused on attending to the business at hand. The way we treat each other seems to be the key. Being with my family. Being connected with people in my community. Challenging abuse in myself and others. Learning even to recognise abuse in a society that is based on abuse. Social justice is still a priority, but I can now see how many of us there are working for that. All I have to do is my bit, not the whole lot. And I have come to see how important it is to be focused on building something rather than attacking something.*

One of the most important things that older lesbians bring to our community is their life experience.

> **LOUISE:** *Being lesbian gave me so much freedom. When I was young you were not allowed to have sex unless you were married. Only a few of my friends lost their virginity before the wedding. You couldn't get contraception. You had to be married to ask a doctor for it. If you were unlucky and got pregnant you got married straight away. Tough shit if you didn't like the bloke. I remember one day after I'd got through all the trauma of accepting that I was a dyke, I realised that I never had to worry about getting pregnant again.*

> **BEV:** *For me, the business of being an older woman is within. And if you come and ask me in twenty years I'll probably give you a different answer. It's a process…*
>
> *As I've grown older I've seen what we are capable of; how tiny our part in this unimaginably huge tapestry of life is. How by industriously stitching away at our own tiny patch we contribute to something that can be beautiful beyond our comprehension – a world free of abuse…I've seen how the most devastating experiences of our lives are the source of our hard-won wisdom. How much there is to learn.*

Older lesbian women have shaped the community that now allows younger lesbians to be out much more easily than in years gone by. Older lesbians have given us the gift of their lives' work. There could easily be an honour roll with many hundreds of women's names on it. Instead, I have the comments of just two:

> **SYLVANA:** *All the bloody hard work we did for years and years! Coming up against the family ethic and having to break through heterosexual society to establish the women's movement – right across the board – and fighting for that*

*and having given so many years of my life to doing that, all
through the 1980s and into the 1990s.*

BEV: *I've taken on some big issues and hard tasks and have
been unswerving in my commitment to these. Racism was
one of those. Social justice was another. I've been a serious
student all my life. I find it lovely to see young women free to
make choices now, which were difficult, or even impossible
for us.*

Sex tips for older dykes

Some of the older lesbians that I spoke to wanted to pass on some sex
tips that they had felt were valuable.

LOUISE: *When you are both older you have to be even more
careful of each other's comfort. You start to think of things
like putting a pillow under her bum for oral sex, to look after
her arthritic hip. You do have to think more about cushions,
lube, that sort of thing. If your partner has arthritis you have
to be very thoughtful about how you do what you do.*

MARIAN: *It's worth debunking the heterosexual myth of the
lesbian sixty-niner. It's bloody difficult to pull off successfully
at any age, and as you get older it's damn near impossible.
Definitely not worth the effort. One position I think should
never be undervalued is where she sits on the edge of the bed
and you kneel between her knees. It's a very workable
position.*

CLAIRE: *It's a reality that I tire more quickly during sex these
days. I think about it and plan round it.*

MARIAN: *You have to cater for less control over various
sphincters. You have to be okay with the odd burp or fart.*

*You have to get your communication up to speed. There are
things like constipation to talk about. If you are with
someone who is only orgasmic with a vibrator you have to
cater for that. You really have to be able to talk to each other
about this kind of thing.*

MENOPAUSE

Dr Christiane Northrup writes that the true meaning of menopause is
a 'coming into' women's wisdom and integrity. It is a time when we can
truly tap into our women-centred power. She argues that menopause is
a coming through, and past, the time when wisdom is cyclic, into a
time when wisdom is steady. In the menstruating years, women's bodies
respond to the cyclic ebb and flow of hormones. With the coming of
menopause, things begin to even out. Concerns change, and the basis
of wisdom becomes more solid.[13] After menopause, a woman is more
likely to live, and speak out, her truth.[14]

There are large numbers of books available on menopause. One of
the best, most balanced, easy to read, accurate and informative
resources that I have found is the chapter on menopause in Christiane
Northrup's work 'Women's Bodies, Women's Wisdom.'[15] Dr Northrup
outlines the physical basis of menopause, looking at the difficulties
which women experience. The chapter also examines Western
medicine treatment options in careful detail, and sets out a range of
herbal, naturopathic, nutritional and holistic alternatives. Some of the
options described in her book are not available in Australia, but this
does not detract from the value of this excellent reference. Dr Christine
Northrup has in 2001 released a new book, entitled *The Wisdom of
Menopause*, in which she expands her views. I don't propose to restate
information that Northrup presents, or which is available from a large
number of other sources.

The approach to menopause that I outline in this section is a very
medical one – this is what I am familiar with. I have not attempted to
present the pros and cons of alternative modalities. My basic stance is

to be respectful of healers from other traditions. As there are many other books on the subject, I will present only a brief overview.

If you are seeking a path through the experience of menopause, I strongly suggest you trust your intuition. There are many alternatives to Western medicine. Yoga, tai chi and other systems, which connect mind and body, can be powerful sources of support and insight. Chinese medicine and acupuncture, homeopathy, herbal medicine and other healing modalities assist many women. Check out the Resource section. Trust your inner wisdom and choose the path that your heart directs you towards.

> **CLAIRE:** *It was a time of huge turmoil, and also of transition, for me. Yes, there were times when I was depressed. Or when I felt irritated by the physical stuff. But I decided take it on as a rite of passage. Just as the hormone surges in adolescence mark a transformation into adulthood, I decided that this marks the passage into the third stage of life. I took time out to look at what was triggering the depression. I made some major changes in my work and relationships. I accepted the hot flushes as the cleansing fires of my own physiology. On my birthday, a year after my last bleeding time, I met with some close women friends to meditate and formally honour the Crone (the archetypal aged woman). I accepted her and welcomed her as part of who I am becoming. And I honoured her as myself.*

The dominant culture sees menopause as a 'deficiency disease'.[16] Large commercial interests have seized the opportunity to market products claimed to remedy its effects.[17] Many advertising campaigns show frail women made young, spry and attractive by whatever product is being promoted. Women must seek their own knowledge and listen to their own intuition to wend their way through the mass of myth and misinformation. It is important that we are not disadvantaged by taking on the dominant culture's view.

Some women experience menopause as the best thing that ever happened to them.

> **LOUISE:** *Menopause has been fantastic for me. I no longer have to worry about bleeding. I always was bossy. I figure that my status as a menopaused woman gives me the right to take no shit, to be listened to, and to be as crusty my mood dictates!*

Many women are not bothered by the physical aspects of menopause. Others experience symptoms that are inconvenient, while a few find them intolerable. Women may note a decline in energy and libido. Some experience hot flushes, or what some choose to define as 'power surges', and rejoice in them. Some also notice vaginal dryness. Women may describe mood swings, depression, anxiety, decreased self-confidence and self-esteem, decreased concentration, forgetfulness, fuzzy thinking and itchy skin. It is important to remember that at the time in her life when she is experiencing menopause, many women face life changes. These may often underpin the psychological symptoms that are attributed to menopause.

It is well documented that the way in which a woman experiences menopause is significantly affected by the cultural context in which she lives.[18] If she expects that there may be problems, then it is much more likely that they will present. If she is from Japan or traditional Navaho Indian culture where menopausal distress is rare, she is likely to pass through the transition without difficulty.[19]

Western women who are experiencing symptoms will often go to their health practitioner to talk about solutions. If a woman goes to a medical practitioner, hormone replacement therapy (HRT) will frequently be offered. Some doctors strongly recommend it for all who are menopausal. I don't agree with the 'all women need to be on it' approach. When I am discussing this issue with a woman, I will ask her history, to find out:

- what the woman is experiencing physically and emotionally;
- whether or not she has had breast cancer or any other cancer; whether she has a family history of these cancers;
- whether she has had heart disease, or a family history of this;

- her history of fractured bones; whether she has a family history of osteoporosis;
- if she smokes, what kind of diet she has and what type and amount of exercise she gets; whether she consumes much caffeine or alcohol;
- whether she has a family history of Alzheimer's disease or dementia, and whether she has been exposed to large amounts of pesticides.

I will also try to find out why the woman is considering HRT. Is it because someone has told her that she should? Is it that she is having difficulty with menopausal symptoms? Or is it because she has heard that it may prevent her having osteoporosis (and broken bones), heart attacks and Alzheimer's disease?

I will also ask about what is going on in her life. Sometimes women think that HRT will solve problems of tiredness, depression or low libido. There are times when life issues need to be addressed instead. If she wants to (and the work setting I am in permits it), I will work with her to identify where her own wisdom leads her on these issues.

Whether or not a woman uses HRT must be her choice. My job as a doctor is to help her weigh up the information presently available about the short- and long-term costs and benefits. My usual advice is: if a woman is not having menopausal symptoms that are unacceptable to her, and if she does not have high risk factors for osteoporosis, then I can see no good reason for her to take HRT, unless for some reason she wants to. If menopausal symptoms or osteoporosis are an issue, then I will help her find a regimen that is suitable for her.

Until very recently, it was believed that HRT protected women from heart disease. Studies released in 2001 cast doubt on this view. Doctors have been advised not to prescribe HRT solely for the purpose of preventing heart attacks and strokes. Studies still in progress will provide more information.[20]

When I'm asked whether HRT protects from dementia I explain that from the evidence presently available, it is not yet possible to give a definite answer to this question. More research is necessary.

Regarding HRT and the risk of breast cancer, I feel that the decision to take HRT should be made by each woman and her doctor only after a very careful consideration of the risks and benefits in each individual's situation. Evidence indicates that there may be no increase in risk of breast cancer with the short-term use of HRT to relieve menopause symptoms. If HRT is used long term there is a definite increase in risk. It is argued that the increase in risk is worth it for the protection from osteoporosis.[21] If a woman has already had breast cancer, or has a strong family history of it, she should discuss this issue with her specialist. Lesbian women may have different risk factors for breast cancer from straight women. Nullparity (having had no children) and increased body size are said to increase the risk of breast cancer. No research has yet adequately addressed this issue.

If the woman is distressed by her experience of menopause and states that she wants to use HRT to see if this will help, then I offer a full gynaecological check-up. I will ensure that her complaint is not caused by thyroid disease, clinical depression or other physical problems. From her history I will determine if there are any reasons why she should not take HRT. These could include high blood pressure that is difficult to control, liver disease or problems with blood clotting.

I will usually have a discussion with her to work out whether it is appropriate to do blood tests to assess hormone levels. Doctors in the United States and some other countries may routinely recommend blood tests, or sometimes saliva or urine tests, to establish hormone levels. Saliva and urine hormone tests are not routinely available in Australia. In this country, many doctors believe that the tests don't give useful information in working out how to deal with menopause. The treatment suggested will depend on the woman's symptoms, not on the result of tests. Therefore, guidelines in this country suggest that blood tests are not usually necessary. The woman's symptoms, and her response to the hormones, are thought to be the best guide to prescribing.

Each individual is different. However, I will often start by suggesting a low dose oestriol or oestradiol, either as a tablet or in a patch or gel absorbed through the skin. Oestrogen may cause the lining of the uterus to grow thicker (endometrial hyperplasia). Occasionally this may be a precursor to cancer. It has been found that this problem is prevented by progestogens. Unless the woman has previously had a hysterectomy, it will be necessary to prescribe a progestogen.

If the woman requests 'natural progesterone', I would explain that in Australia, this is not approved as an alternative to progestogen. 'Natural progesterone' is made in a laboratory from hormones found in plants (mostly yams and soybeans). These hormones are modified so that they are identical to the progesterone made in women's bodies. They are sometimes called 'bioidentical hormones'. Some theorists argue that if HRT is required, then 'natural progesterone' is the substance of choice.[22] Accepted clinical evidence has not yet demonstrated that this prevents endometrial hyperplasia and decreased bone density in the same way that synthetic progestogens do.[23] If the woman still requests it, after a discussion of the risks and benefits, I would prescribe a 'natural' progesterone cream compounded by a reputable pharmacist. If a woman chose this course of action I would advise her to have regular checks to ensure that she did not develop endometrial hyperplasia or other cancers.

Hormone replacement often requires two or three months of treatment before its effect can be assessed. It sometimes takes several adjustments to find the right combination for an individual woman. If the main problem is reduced libido or reduced energy, and an oestrogen/progestogen (or progesterone) combination does not provide relief, I may discuss the use of testosterone with the client. Testosterone has not been approved in Australia for this use; however, some women and their doctors have found that small doses may dramatically improve libido and energy levels.

If the woman's concern is vaginal dryness or recurrent urinary tract infections I would advise her to consider a vaginal oestrogen cream or pessary. Often, a direct application of cream is far more effective than any other type of hormone replacement for these problems.

If the woman is concerned about osteoporosis, and would not otherwise be considering HRT, I will often suggest that she have a bone density scan. If the bone density scan is normal I advise on diet, weight-bearing exercise and mineral and vitamin supplements. I suggest that she repeats the scan in two years' time. Only if her bone density is dropping do I advise her to consider HRT.

For many of the problems discussed above, there are solutions offered by health care workers from non-medical modalities. Many of the treatments are practical and useful. Some are not. The choice of therapy will depend on the individual woman, her needs and her background.

It should be remembered that I started my account of my medical approach to menopause with the words: 'If the woman is distressed by her experience of menopause'. Large numbers of woman are unworried by ' the change'. Many are empowered by it! Some embrace 'the change' as a time to reclaim themselves and their power.

Some see menopause as a time of new beginnings.

> **LOUISE:** *I feel it's important for women to remember that their lives are in their own hands. As lesbians we may often choose to do things differently. So you have lesbian women having their Croning celebrations to give sacred space to their coming 'of age'. And you have women who do not choose to use Western medicine. I think it is important to remember the deep and wide power of connection with other women, and to remember the usefulness of self-help groups. Women's Health Centres exist, we can use them. Institutions often see that ageing women equals medical menopause. But we can use their resources to set up our own networks and to get our needs met by each other.*

> **CLAIRE:** *Menopause was a gateway to that time of life when all that I had worked for came together. I have learned who I am. I know what I want in life. I have the confidence to go after it. I finally feel sure of myself and of my own wisdom.*

14

Doubly Difficult

Some women have absolutely no difficulty in finding, accepting and integrating their lesbian identity. Others experience profound trauma. Many factors influence what the process will be like. These may include the personality and personal style of the lesbian woman, and also her family and cultural background. For some, there are additional issues that make acceptance of lesbian sexuality much more difficult. I am not able to speak for the many who have had a much harder time than me. It is important that they have space to speak for themselves.

J is a lesbian woman. Her cultural background is Korean. She has lived in Australia for eight years. She put her experience in a nutshell for me.

> **J:** *Sometimes I feel like I live within the prison of people's perception. My family has very set, old-fashioned values. The way I am seen by people who don't know me is as a meek little Asian girl. The commands of my culture are so rigid; they are like iron bars. I constantly feel that I have to be vigilant, to go after what I want. I always know that when I go against my family culture to follow my heart, I am doing*

it at a big cost. You have to look deep within yourself, past the layers and layers of other people's perceptions, to find out who you really are. I feel that our difficulty in being ourselves is more than doubled.

Aboriginal lesbians

CATHERINE: *No-one in my family had ever heard of the word lesbian. It was a completely alien concept. Occasionally they did talk about 'poofters' but it was seen totally as a white man's disease. I have not even considered coming out to my family.*

DONNA: *At lesbian events you have to deal with racism. At home with your family you have to deal with homophobia. Where can I be at ease? Where can I just be all of who I am?*

Lesbians from non-English speaking backgrounds

GINA: *I have contact with my family. But they absolutely will not tolerate my partner. My relationship is never talked about. My partner is not welcome at my parents' home. And on the other hand, I don't fit fully into the lesbian community. I have some wonderful women friends but there are some things about me they will never understand.*

Catholic lesbians

RAY: *A day doesn't go by without me feeling the agony of the split. The church is a huge part of my daily life. It is in every part of my thinking and breathing. They tell me that being a lesbian is depraved. And yet after years of struggling with it, I know that I really am lesbian. I also know, to the depths of my being, that God loves me and doesn't care. But there is always the guilt. That Catholic baggage. Every day is just unsolvable emotional turmoil.*

Christian, Buddhist, Hindu and Jewish women have also spoken to me about their struggles with similar issues. Any religion or culture that is intolerant of difference can be the cause of deep distress.

Mental illness

LILLIAN: *You are always hiding. There are always two coming out decisions. I'd accepted my lesbian identity and sorted coming out as a dyke. Then I got the diagnosis of bi-polar disorder. You are 'in the closet' with that too. There is always shame. You have to come to terms with it and accept yourself. And then there is each and every decision of whether to tell the people you are mixing with. In some ways, having come out as a dyke before, I knew that process. I won't say it's made it easier. But at least I know the process of having to weigh up on each occasion: is this a safe person to tell? And usually, it's not that I'm gay that I'm thinking about.*

Physical disability

TONIA: *When you are in a wheelchair, lots of people only see the wheelchair. They do not see the dyke. They often do not make eye contact with you. They certainly do not see you as a sexual being. You already have trouble with body image. I mean you really have to get over it to see yourself as attractive. You do not fit the cultural norm for what is attractive. I think I do all right with that. I believe that I am an attractive person. What I have so much difficulty with is when people just don't recognise that I have any sexuality at all. Their astonished reactions when they get to know I'm going to a dyke event.*

YVONNE: *I have Crohn's disease and I had a bowel resection when I was 17. It left me with a stoma – a bag on my stomach that collects my poo. Try that when you are just starting up a new relationship. Think about what it's like* *when you are going out with a person. You look normal in your clothes. You have to work out how they will react before you are in bed. You have to talk about it in advance. I have had women react with absolute disgust, or treat me like I was a freak.*

CYNTHIA: *I am a carrier of Hep B. It can be transmitted by my saliva. I can't even share an apple with anyone. I have to choose between not telling people at all (and putting them at risk of getting it too), telling them (and maybe getting rejected), or just never having sex. Basically my sex life is completely stuffed.*

Intellectual disability

BRIANA: *It can be difficult and uncomfortable for parents or carers to accept that a person with an intellectual disability has a sexual relationship at all, let alone consider that it may be with a same-sex partner. People who work with intellectually disabled clients can also find this confronting. In recent years there has been some change in attitude and a realisation of the need to educate people with developmental disabilities, so courses about personal development and sexuality have been introduced. The Disability Act is about the rights of people with disabilities having the same choices as everyone, including the sexual relationship of their choice.*

OPPRESSION

Women have talked to me about the grief, fear, frustration and anger associated with many problems that are both obvious and invisible. Difference, whether physical or cultural, visible or imperceptible, may give rise to emotional as well as tangible disconnection from others.

Women may feel alienated when an important part of themselves is both unrecognised and considered by others to be shocking or unacceptable. This is the very same reaction that many lesbian women have faced in relation to their sexual identity. When a problem is invisible the woman may feel that she herself is negated. Mastectomy, HIV infection, chronic fatigue syndrome, severe arthritis and back pain are just a few of the physical difficulties that are not easily visible.

When the difference is readily perceptible, women often feel that those around them react only in ways governed by stereotyping beliefs that relate to their difference, rather than to the woman as a person.

Society as a whole tacitly agrees on what constitutes acceptable behaviour and appearance. And yet the norm, the 'dominant story' is an illusion. Very few people actually conform to it. Privately, most people have at least one aspect of themselves around which they feel a sense of being different from others, of 'not fitting in'. We have all been hoodwinked by the myth that there is a state of being which is 'normal'.

Groups will often ostracise or victimise anyone who does not conform to their norms. This can be conscious and deliberate oppression, or it can be careless words or thoughtless lashing out. Acts of oppression are often based in fear and insecurity. People make themselves feel bigger or safer by picking on others. Acts of oppression may also be based in greed or power-seeking.

Sometimes oppressive actions are based on behaviour patterns that have been acquired through the oppressor's own history as a victim of abuse. When a person has been a victim of severe abuse, it may be difficult for them to work out what kind of behaviour is acceptable and what is abusive. People who have been victims of long-term abuse may receive further mistreatment and be unable to identify that the behaviour directed towards them is not acceptable. In turn, their feelings may be so numb, and their awareness so blunted, that they do not perceive the impact of their own abusive actions.

Our culture has come to a point where oppression is seen as absolutely unacceptable. We are encouraged to look at our own fears and to deal with them in ways that do not harm others. Individuals are expected to be aware of the impact of their behaviour patterns on others. If conduct could damage others, our culture now directs that we must choose different actions. More and more often, we are seeing oppression named, confronted and stopped.

As a lesbian community we are mindful that we have been marginalised, excluded from mainstream culture. Many of us feel a responsibility to actively oppose cruelty and persecution. We need to be ever vigilant that our community itself does not oppress minority groups.

The issues that women confront in their lives may separate them from mainstream culture. They may also result in feelings that it's very difficult to meet other lesbians. There may be physical problems like difficulty of access to venues with wheelchairs. Asian women have said that they feel that nightclubs and dances are just too threatening.[1] Women from non-English speaking backgrounds may feel that cultural and language barriers make it difficult for them to be part of the lesbian community.[2] Although the lesbian community has a long feminist history of being actively inclusive, it may at times seem to be unfriendly.[3] Structures are not in place at every venue or at every gathering to help women to feel comfortable and to meet others.

> **TONIA:** *What has helped me create lesbian friendships and relationships? Communication first up! You have to say what you need. It's hard at the best of times, but if you want to create connection, you have to say it. Also, accepting who I am. Accepting the loss of mobility. Accepting the absolutely rooted body image. Accepting how bloody angry I am about that, and the grief. And with all that, deciding that I am still a good person. I am still an attractive person! I think a lot has had to do with my attitude, just going for it. And just getting on with it.*

Our community is 'non-homogenous'.[4] Lesbians are vastly disparate in their politics, class, financial status, family structure, relationship patterns, ethnicity and culture. It can be difficult to locate people who are like-minded. (However, this is true for people of every sexual orientation.) It is difficult enough at times being lesbian, but it is more than doubly difficult having another major difference to contend with.

There are no words that express an adequate response to this truth. It is important to acknowledge the extreme hardship that many women face in the journeys of their lives. We must not deny their stories. We must educate ourselves and act in ways that contribute to making their journeys easier.

Running through most of our organisations and communities there is an awareness of our need to connect across our diversity. We choose not to replicate mainstream structures and systems that perpetuate abuse. Rather we attempt to develop systems of relating to each other which are based on inclusion and equality. We have not got it right. We are constantly finding ways in which our organisations and communities need to adjust and improve.

15

Lesbian Courage

I t takes courage to identify as lesbian. A woman has to be prepared to acknowledge that within her there are thoughts and feelings which some in the dominant culture still find unacceptable. It takes even more courage to name the difference 'lesbian', 'dyke', 'gay', 'queer', 'bi' or 'transgender'. It takes further huge courage to come out and acknowledge your identity to friends, family and community.

A selection process takes place. Every woman who identifies as lesbian was either a woman of courage from the outset or has acquired courage in the course of determining her lesbian identity. The necessity to confront these issues, and find her way in the world, demands this. Her courage may be of the quiet, careful type, the brave, bold type, or something in between. If she names her identity, or acts on her lesbian feelings, then courage exists within her.

When making decisions about her lesbian identity, each woman has choices. She may ignore her lesbian identity. She may acknowledge it, but remain 'in the closet', hiding her truth from those around her. Or she may choose to come out. In the past, only very brave souls chose to be open. The choice to be 'out' is much more available to women today.

This selection process has had results. Many lesbian women of courage have taken things into their own hands. They've changed their lives. They've changed their families and communities. Lesbians have helped to influence culture and public policy both in Australia and in the world.

The structure of lesbian families may have contributed to their capacity to do this. While other family structures exist, couples are the most common arrangement. If the lesbian family consists of partners with children, both adults may have skills and interest in child-care. A large number of lesbian women are in partnerships and do not have children. Many lesbian women choose to remain single. Some have rejected the concept of family; others embrace it.

If the lesbian household consists of women who both work, each may be familiar with the demands of a career. They will often support each other in order to meet goals. This is not at all uncommon in heterosexual relationships. However, until recently there has been a culturally based assumption that the man's career would come first, and that he would be the 'breadwinner'. This notion has not entirely disappeared in Western culture.

As a result of their family structures, lesbian women have been freer than their heterosexual sisters to devote time and energy to employment, art, literature and other pursuits outside the home. This has meant that some have reached positions of influence in business, government and the arts, although many lesbians were forced by prudence to remain closeted. Nevertheless, while they may not have been visible, their influence has been felt.

Lesbian visibility began in Australia in 1970. 'Australia's first openly homosexual political organisation' was a women-only group, Daughters of Bilitis (after the American organisation of the same name).[1] The founders were Marion Paull and Claudia Pearce.[2] In the same year Christabel Poll (and her friend John Ware) were interviewed for a feature article about homosexual relationships by a national newspaper, The Australian.[3] The story went to press on 19 September 1970.[4] This was a first in Australia.

In 1972 Clover Club began to have meetings. This social club for lesbian women held regular Friday night get-togethers for many years. Clover acquired its own club rooms in Drummoyne, Sydney. While these premises have since been sold, the group has continued to exist and provide social enjoyment for members to the present time.

In 1973 Radicalesbians formed in Melbourne. While short-lived, this group had a profound and long-lived political impact. Many in this group were lesbian separatists. This philosophy includes a view that women can only truly escape oppression in complete separation from men. A group set out to pursue this aim. In 1974 lesbians collectively purchased a tract of land on the mid-north coast of New South Wales. Subsequently, additional 'women's lands' were established at other locations. Many women (including this author) have had their horizons enriched and broadened by the lives and politics of the women from the lands. Artists, authors, academics, businesswomen, public sector managers and employees have issued from these groups of women. They continue to have their impact in Australian politics today.

Lesbian political activism is based on an opposition to the politics of oppression. Lesbian organisations saw a need to develop their own internal structures and management systems, intended to counter the injustice inherent in mainstream institutions.

HELEN: *In those early days our organisations were collectives – egalitarian, not hierarchical. Our decisions were by consensus. Meetings were facilitated, not chaired. Everybody had her say. Every point of view was valued. There was space for all, no matter how inarticulate a woman might have been. We all took responsibility to ensure that women who had difficulty with words were supported to have a voice. If it appeared a woman might be hurt by the process, we looked after her.*

Now I look around at some of the methods in the organisation where I work. They come from the same base. The other day an employee had a traumatic incident. I automatically contacted him to offer counselling. I know that other groups like the Conflict Resolution Network and Quakers developed these methods. But I know some of the women who introduced these practices to my workplace. And

*I know that they got them from our old activist days. I see
our meeting methods written about in 'new-age' management
manuals. And I smile to see the flow-on effect we have had.*

Courageous women came out and began businesses to serve the lesbian
population. Dawn O'Donnell managed Ruby's (a Sydney nightclub)
from 1976 to 1986.[5] *Lesbians on the Loose* (LOTL) credits her with
'...almost single-handedly creating gay nightlife in Sydney in the
1960s'.[6] Dawn was also involved in a large number of other Sydney
business enterprises.[7]

From the early 1970s, women began to establish commercial
ventures aimed at attracting women-centred women as consumers. At
first there were just a few businesses. Helen-the-printer produced
'women-inspired jewellery'; Wildwise advertised adventures for
women. A permaculture design course for women was established. A
vast array of women in business are now advertising for women clients.
These include: alternative health practitioners, accommodation
enterprises, antique furniture, cafés, caterers, civil celebrants for
commitment ceremonies, counsellors, electricians, escort and dating
services, financiers, framing services, hairdressers, home delivery fruit
and vegetables, insurance brokers, Internet service providers, jewellery
designers and retailers, lawn mowers, mechanics, night spots, nurseries
and garden centres, optometrists, pet grooming services, pharmacists,
publishers, pushbike retailers and manufacturers, psychics, real estate
agents, removalists, sex shops, sex toy retailers, solicitors, tarot readers,
therapists, travel agents, veterinarians and website designers.

Bookshops became meeting places for women. These included The
Feminist Bookshop in Sydney, Murphy Sisters in Adelaide, Shrew in
Melbourne, Arcane Bookshop in Perth and the Brisbane Women's
Bookshop. They led the field in their respective states. Others followed.

In 1984 Lavender and Judith Haggard provided the spark that
started *Lesbian Network*, Australia's only national lesbian newsletter.
This publication for 'womin-identified wimmin only' was (and still is)
aimed at strengthening lesbian culture. It provided a bridge between
feminist and non-feminist lesbians. True to its name, the publication
has kept women informed of national events and community news

from that time until the present day. It publishes original articles, letters, artworks and poetry.

In the various states, local women's newsletters were springing up. Examples included Perth's *Grapevine* and Newcastle's *No Frills*, the latter of which was started by a small group in 1988. It eventually folded but other Newcastle newsletters followed. The process that occurred here was repeated Australia-wide; the work of one group inspired women in another location. For example, a *Grapevine* reader who had moved from Perth to the east coast was the prime mover for the Newcastle magazine. These newsletters were frequently directed to the women's community generally. However, lesbian energy fuelled the enterprises. Lesbian women were often the primary volunteer workforce. These newsletters were a means of advertising lesbian events and had a large lesbian readership.

Frances Rand and Jaz Ishtar decided that a 'What's On' for Sydney dykes was needed. They established 'Lesbians on the Loose'. The first edition was published in January 1990. It was eight pages long and hand-made. Frances Rand nurtured LOTL through to it present form, a glossy publication with a circulation of 20,000 Australia-wide.[8]

There were several national lesbian gatherings in the 1970s and 1980s. Regular events began in 1989, with the National Lesbian Conference and Celebration held in January of that year. This was followed by the First National Lesbian Conference, held in Melbourne in 1990. The Lesbian Space Project ('LSP') received its first broad public hearing in the same year.[9] This ambitious project began when Australian lesbians were challenged to donate $250,000 within a period of one year. The target was met and a building purchased to house the lesbian space. By the end of 1993, project supporters were divided over the issue of inclusion of transgender people (who defined themselves as lesbian). Those involved were unable to resolve this issue. The building was subsequently sold.

In 1991 a group of lesbians took a huge risk and hired the Sydney Opera House Concert Hall for a concert entitled 'Living Our Passion'. It featured out lesbians: Robyn Archer, Deborah Cheetham, Judy Small, comic Sue-Anne Post and the Top Twins.[10] The Concert Hall was crammed!

CAROL: *I went to that concert and walked away from the Opera House afterwards in an absolute state of euphoria that so many dykes could be in one public place at one time.*

At music festivals and women's concerts we 'winced and laughed' at songs about lesbian life by Barbara David, Sue Edmonds and others.[11] Women's music was supported by the 'Wimmin's Music Network' and women's music festivals. Imports included the unforgettable Alex Dobkin, who toured Australia several times. Groups committed to bringing lesbian music to lesbians included 'Prodyketions' and later 'Lavender Music'.

The Women's Circus was launched in Melbourne in 1991. The Circus aimed to reaffirm women's control over their own bodies and build self-esteem through physical and performance work.[12] POW (Powerful Old Women) was a part of this circus.

The Women's Library was also established in Sydney in 1991. The *Journal of Australian Lesbian Feminist Studies* (an initiative of the Lesbian Studies and Research Group) was also published for the first time.[13]

Lesbian culture and women's culture flourished in conferences, 'confests', 'ovulars', concerts, women's spirituality weekends, women's camps, womyns festivals, LesFests, lesbian studies weekends, ongoing discussion groups, 'consciousness raising' groups, 'coming out' groups, social groups, support groups, religious and political groups. Aboriginal lesbians formed The Koori Wirguls, Asian Lesbians formed Sydney Asian Lesbians. In 1981 a Gay and Lesbian Business Association was established in Sydney. Similar groups were soon established in other states.[14]

On the international scene, The Michigan Womyn's Music Festival was first held in August 1976. Meg Christian, Alex Dobkin and Chris Williamson, described as the 'foremothers of lesbian music', have been out since the Seventies; kd lang has been a lesbian icon for years. Melissa Etheridge came out in 1995 at President Clinton's Inauguration Ball.[15] Ellen DeGeneres said 'Yep, I'm Gay' on the front cover of *Time* in April 1997.[16]

In science, lesbian women have had their impact. It has not always been acknowledged. Dr Beverly Whipple and Dr John Perry told the world about the G spot at a meeting of the Society for the Scientific Study of Sex in 1980. They released their book *The G Spot* in 1983. Additional background is set out by the authors of *A New View of a Woman's Body*:

> A group of lesbians, having had this experience (of ejaculation), related their observations to sex researchers Beverly Whipple, R. N. and John Perry Ph.D. In reviewing the literature, Whipple and Perry found that a researcher named Grafenberg had reported similar findings in the early 1950s...'[17]

Perry and Whipple went on to write and release their book.

The Coalition for Activist Lesbians (COAL), was established in 1994 to work for lesbian visibility and human rights. This organisation was the only specifically lesbian organisation with delegates accredited to be present at the United Nations World Conference on Women, held in Beijing in 1995; 198 countries had delegates in attendance. COAL has also received major Australian mainstream recognition. In December 1996 the group received a $95,000 grant from the NSW State Government to produce 'Out For Action', a high-quality kit 'aimed at new and emerging lesbians to provide information about lesbian identity, lesbian culture and community and human rights'.[18]

In Australian politics, it wasn't until 1995 that Susan Harben was 'the first out lesbian to be preselected by a major party to contest the NSW state election...'[19] In 1996, Australia's 'first out dyke politician...Greens Senator Giz Watson romped home in the Legislative Council elections in WA' (Western Australia).[20] Giz made a deliberate decision to be open about her sexuality and made it clear that she was prepared to work for lesbian and gay law reform before the election.[21]

In the Uniting Church there had been years of haggling over whether homosexuals should be accepted.[22] In July 1997 the Rev Dorothy McRae-McMahon, then aged 63, '... stood up in front of 500 delegates to the National Assembly and declared herself a lesbian'.[23]

There was a high cost. She received letters that contained vitriol like 'Dear Filth...'[24] Two charges of misconduct were laid against her. She survived both and retained her ordination. By October 1997 Rev McRae-McMahon nevertheless felt it necessary to resign her senior position within the church. 'Until her resignation in September as Director of Mission, Dorothy was the second-most senior figure in the Uniting Church. Her work for social justice earned her the Human Rights Medal and a United Nations Peace Prize.'[25]

Also in 1997, Lisa-Marie Vizaniari, Australia's hope for a medal in the discus at the Sydney 2000 Olympics, made a deliberate choice to come out. She hoped that her openness might provide a role model for other women. She was the first female Olympian ever to openly acknowledge her lesbian identity.[26] Another great sportswoman had previously paved the way – Martina Navratilova had delighted lesbians since she came out in the 1980s.

In February 1998 Kerryn Phelps, a well-known medical practitioner and media commentator married her partner Jacqui Stricker. (They requested that the word 'marriage' rather than 'commitment ceremony' be used in reference to their pledge to each other.)[27] Against their wishes, they were outed by the *Daily Telegraph*. In the print media, columnist Mike Gibson viciously attacked their right to marry.[28] This did not prevent Kerryn subsequently being elected to the position of President of the Australian Medical Association (NSW).

In July 1999 the First Annual Australian National Lesbian Doctors Conference was held. The 19 doctors who attended went on to form ALMA (the Australian Lesbian Medical Association), which now has over a hundred doctors on its mailing list. Australian lesbians lawyers, teachers and vets have formed associations.

Lesbians have fought (and continue to fight) for equal access to fertility clinics. JM, a woman who commenced a legal battle against one of Queensland's clinics, acknowledged that the process was extremely stressful.[29] Lesbians have challenged the status quo by taking large Australian corporations who have discriminated against them to court.[30] Lesbian and gay organisations have successfully lobbied for law reform and continue to push for equal rights in all states and in relation to all matters. Major areas of inequality still exist.

All this history has had an effect. As lesbians have had the courage to be visible, it has become safer and safer for others to make a choice to come out. A large number of organisations now target the 'lavender dollar' with their advertising: Toyota, Telstra, Ella Baché and Qantas are just a few.

There are all types of lesbian courage. Some women have been change agents for the culture. Others find the changes occurring in themselves and their families.

> **CLAIRE:** *I saw one of the most courageous things ever, only a couple of months ago. A young friend of mine told her mother she was a dyke. Her mother replied if that was the case, she could not live at home. My friend said, 'Mum, if you stick by that, you'll lose me'. There are people for whom there is no choice, my friend was one – she had the guts to insist on the right to be is who she is. She was prepared to lose her mother. It didn't happen that way, but it could have. That is courage to me.*

Despite all the changes and the increased acceptance in our culture, lesbian women still suffer from discrimination and victimisation as a result of our sexual orientation.

Each one of us who comes out makes the world safer for every lesbian, dyke, bi, transgender or queer woman who follows. Our existence also forces the culture we live in to examine and re-examine its attitudes towards tolerance, and its acceptance of diversity.

> **BEV:** *We can never assume that once the gains have been made they will not be overthrown. Look at the 'policies' of One Nation! All it takes is a change of government! We have to be eternally vigilant!*

Appendix 1:
Approaches to Orgasm

This appendix is for women who do not have orgasms as often as they would like, or in the way that they would like, or who have never had an orgasm at all.

First, ensure that you are familiar with the contents of Chapter 7, 'Orgasm', and the section titled 'Difficulty with orgasm' in Chapter 8.

If you are having difficulties with orgasm, ask yourself a few questions: do you get aroused but don't have orgasms? Do you find that you just don't get aroused? (If so, see 'Problems with desire', p. 101). Have you explored your body? Are you comfortable with sexual activity? Have you felt that you would have an orgasm if only she would keep on doing it to you long enough? Do you give yourself enough time to climax? Or do you lie there thinking 'I'd better come soon or she's going to get bored/jaw ache/whatever'?

In this Appendix, I have set out a number of suggestions that you may like to consider. These will not be useful for all women. If you feel inclined to try a suggestion, do so. If you are not attracted to a particular activity, ignore it. Trust your intuition and adopt only the suggestions that appeal to you.

The essentials

- Give yourself enough time. Some women can take more than an hour of stimulation to reach orgasm.
- Strengthen your pubococcygeus muscle. Studies have indicated that increasing the strength of your pelvic floor can lead to increased orgasmic capacity. Appendix 2 sets out exercises that can assist (p. 215).
- Identify and address any relationship issues that you feel may be getting in the way.
- Get what you want. Some women need to be stimulated in very specific ways to come to orgasm. This is okay! If you suspect that this is true for you, invest the time and energy to find out exactly what you need.
- Learn to communicate really well.

> **LOUISE**: *I really had to get to the point where I could say to Ellie, 'I can only come when I can sit on your face and see you lick my cunt and clit'. It's partly the visual thing that does it for me. I was scared that she'd think I was too weird, or that she wouldn't want to do it. But we were just going nowhere with orgasm for me till I was able to ask her.*

- Masturbate. Explore your own sensuality. Whether absent orgasm is primary or secondary, one of the very best ways of addressing it is through masturbation. It's a great way of learning about yourself and becoming comfortable with all sorts of sexual practices. Fantasy may also be useful. Be prepared to try new things. Re-read Chapter 6 and set lots of private time aside to masturbate.

- Buy a vibrator. Many women come to orgasm through no other means than with a vibrator. There is nothing abnormal or wrong about this. It just means you need more rhythmic and stronger stimulation than a human can provide. Vibrators can be used for self-satisfaction or in partner sex. Bless the Goddess for the fact that we live in a technological age, and go for it!

- Masturbate with your partner. If the only way you can come to orgasm is by masturbation, that's fine! One of the good things about being a lesbian is that we have redefined sex. Anything that feels like sex is sex! Masturbating while another person watches or participates in some way that is acceptable to you and non-intrusive can be very intimate. It can also be very confronting to take part in masturbation with another person. You can open yourself and your soul when masturbating with another person watching, as much as in sex where you physically entwine. If you are the person masturbating, you allow yourself to be seen. You may be open and vulnerable. You may delight in putting on a sensual show. If you are the person watching, you are being present for one of the most intimate of human activities. The connection can be profound. Or the erotic experience can be exquisite. Or both.

- Tune in to yourself and your own sensations. The essence of experiencing orgasm is being able to perceive and enjoy the feelings that are occurring in your body. (See 'Sensate focus for lesbians' below.)

- Stay positive. There is a very common vicious cycle: you think you won't have an orgasm, so you don't, so your expectations are reinforced. Don't get into that one! It truly is important to let the focus of sexual activity be sensual pleasure and intimacy, not orgasm. Really delight in the enjoyment that is available.

- Consider the idea that becoming orgasmic is a journey. It is about claiming your own pleasure and your sensual power. You may learn lots about yourself on the journey. Like all journeys worth travelling, it may take some time.

Sensate focus for lesbians

The classic method of dealing with absent orgasm is 'sensate focus'. It is old, but it is effective. It was first described by Masters and Johnston for heterosexuals in 1966.

Many authors have presented variations of this technique. The method works by asking you change your goals when you have sex. Instead of orgasm being your aim, you are asked to allow your focus to be enjoyment instead. It can be used in conjunction with a therapist, or as a self-help tool.

Preliminaries

If you are using this Appendix as a self-help tool, I would ask you first to have a discussion with your partner about orgasm. Do this in a room that you do not usually have sex in. If you normally make love in the bedroom, have this discussion in the living room. Talk about your sexual likes and dislikes. Tell her if there are things that turn you on. Tell her if there is anything that turns you off. Try to state as clearly as possible any problems that you are aware of that stand in the way of sexual enjoyment. If you find it difficult to talk about these things, then each of you write three lists setting out the sexual activities you like, the sexual activities you don't like, and the sexual activities that are difficult for you. Then share these lists with each other.

Next, reach an agreement to set some time aside for sexual activity. Mark the times on the calendar or put them in your diary, just like you would for any other appointment that is important to you. You will need at least four sessions of two hours each. You can decide the frequency. Once a week? More often? Once a fortnight? (I wouldn't make them any farther apart than that.) You may need several sessions of two hours at each of the stages set out below.

Create privacy. If necessary, employ a babysitter or send the kids to their grandparents for the evening.

Make a commitment to spend time on your sex life. Don't let anything get in the way. You may find it interesting to note the sort of things that will arise which will tempt you not to keep your appointments with each other. Don't let them. Your sex life is more important.

When you get to your appointment with each other, lock the doors and take the phone off the hook.

Do not be fooled into thinking that you can skip any of the sessions.

Stage One

The first step is for you to take turns touching each other.

At this stage, you are instructed not to touch the intimate erogenous zones (genitals, anus and breasts). It is intended that the touch is not sexual in nature.

First, one woman touches and the other is passive, and then you reverse roles. Put a clock somewhere so that you will know when to swap. Each person should be in each role for at least half an hour (preferably 45 minutes).

The woman who is doing the touching should caress and explore the body of the other for her own interest and pleasure. She is not to try and please her partner, but to touch as she chooses. She should notice what surfaces and textures she likes to touch. Where does she like to put her fingers and lips? Notice if you move to pleasuring your partner, and move back to pleasuring yourself!

The receiver should focus on her own sensations. She may use either verbal or non-verbal communication to let her partner know if she does not like something. Her awareness should be on her own sensations, perceptions and feelings.

Let the sessions be without words. The silence minimises distraction from the sensations.

If you feel turned on and think you are going to have an orgasm, back off! Change what you are doing. Cool down! Orgasm is not permitted at this stage of the process.

After each woman has been in each role, talk about what happened. Talk about your feelings and fears.

Stage Two

Go on to Stage Two when you both feel ready to. This may be on your second appointment with each other, or it may be after several appointments at Stage One.

Again you take turns to touch and receive. At this stage, more intimate touch is allowed. Each session starts with the non-genital areas and should stay with non-sexual touch for some time. However, touch that includes breasts, genitals and anus is permitted. Neither penetration nor orgasms are permitted.

The active woman is still asked to touch for her own pleasure.

The receiver is asked to concentrate on what she would like, and to communicate this non-verbally. You may like to use a technique called 'hand riding'. The receiver puts her hand on her partner's hand. Non-verbally she indicates how she would like what her partner is doing to change. She can also show her partner what she wants. She may convey that she prefers lighter touch, more pressure, faster or slower strokes or to change the place where she is being touched. The session should still, as far as possible, be silent.

After each partner has had a turn in each role, talk about what happened. Do not move on to Stage Three until you both feel comfortable to do so. Have as many appointments as you need at Stage Two.

Stage Three

Again, take the phone off the hook and lock the doors.

In this stage, the touching is mutual. You are asked to go from the obviously artificial taking of turns, to a more natural exchange of touch. Shift your attention away from just your own sensations and bring it to the interaction that is going on between you. Penetration and orgasm are still prohibited. If either partner becomes so aroused that orgasm seems imminent, stop and return to non-genital touching. The aim is still to explore sensation and pleasure. Orgasm is definitely not the goal.

Stage Four

The fourth stage is a session of mutual touch, including if the receiver wishes it, touching inside the entrance of the vagina or anus. You are allowed to ride up to the edge of orgasm but not cross over.

If you feel that orgasm is imminent, back off. Change what you are doing.

When the session is over, talk about what happened for each of you.

By the time that you have had several sessions at Stage Four, many women find that they have no difficulty proceeding to climax.

Appendix 2:
Applied Anatomy

In this appendix I have provided additional information about two subjects which are vitally important to women's sexual enjoyment: the G spot, and pelvic floor exercises.

The G spot

Whether or not the G spot exists has been a matter of contention. Whether women ejaculate has also been hotly debated. There are thousands of women who need no convincing about these issues. Many women know that when they have a full bladder they may feel sexually pleasurable sensations in their vulva and lower abdomen, even in the absence of touch or stimulation. Sexual activity with a full bladder can be enormously pleasurable. Any woman who has experienced this knows that the urethra has sexual significance. Dr Helen O'Connell's recent work lends academic support to this view.

The 'G spot' is the name given to the area on the vaginal wall that overlies the tissue that surrounds the urethra. It was named after the physician who described it (Grafenberg, in 1950). Feminists have called it the urethral sponge.[1] Dr Helen O'Connell calls it simply 'surrounding erectile tissue'.[2] It is intrinsically linked with the clitoris. See the diagram on p. 26.

The arguments don't matter. Two things are certain:

- Stimulating the spot (whatever it is comprised of) is extremely pleasurable for many women.
- Some women emit fluid when they have orgasms. They are more likely to do this when the G spot is stimulated. There can be a little bit of fluid or a lot. The nature of the fluid has still not been determined. However, releasing fluid is one of the normal things that can happen at orgasm.

The G spot is on the inside of the vagina, on the anterior (front) wall, about five centimetres inside. The G spot is the erectile tissue that surrounds the urethra. Stimulating it can make you feel like urinating. If you're going to explore, urinate first (that way, you won't have to act on the urge if it arises).

Sitting or squatting, use your fingers and explore the inside front wall of the vagina. Use firm upward and outward pressure. You may use one finger or two. The area is about two-thirds of the length of your finger inside. Some women put pressure on the abdomen just above their pubic bone with their other hand. Stroking from inside, in an upwards (ie that is, towards your abdomen) direction, you may feel a pad of tissue under the surface of the vaginal wall. When stimulated it may become firmer. It is important to realise that the G spot responds to deep, firm pressure. The G spot does not respond to light touch. This is one of the reasons, it is believed, that it was not discovered by medical researchers. Doctors are not permitted to touch their patients in this way.

The G spot can be found while lying on your back. However, many women find it a bit awkward to locate in this position. Our arms aren't quite long enough. It's easier to find while sitting or squatting. Once you are familiar with it, though, you'll be able to locate it while lying down. It's also easy to stimulate your partner's G spot. A very effective way is to place one hand on her lower abdomen, just above her pubic bone. Place a finger or two inside her and stroke deeply and firmly stroke along the urethra, towards you.

Women report that when they have orgasms as a result of stimulating this spot, the orgasms are different in nature from orgasms from clitoral manipulation. You will find that some vibrators are specially designed to stimulate the spot.

The puboccygeal muscles (pelvic floor)

The vitally important puboccygeal muscles are the muscles that make up the pelvic floor. The puboccygeus muscle is a multi-layer muscle that stretches like a sling (or hammock) from the coccyx (the tailbone) to the pubic bone (that hard bone you can feel just above your pubic mound. There are three openings in the pelvic floor: the urethra (through which urine flows to the outside), the vagina, and the anus.

A very simple diagram is shown below:

Pelvic floor exercises are sometimes called 'Kegels', after Dr Arnold Kegel, who described the exercises, and asserted that a strong pelvic floor increases sexual satisfaction.

Why bother strengthening your pelvic floor?

A strong pelvic floor can enhance sexual pleasure and increase capacity for orgasm. It has a good chance of helping control urinary incontinence (the embarassing tendency to wet yourself when you cough, or sneeze, or just can't get to the toilet in time). If you might be pregnant in the future, ability to control your pelvic floor muscles may assist with relaxation during labour. Strong muscles also heal more rapidly if they are torn during delivery. A strong pubococcygeus can help prevent pelvic organ prolapse. Prolapse occurs when a woman's uterus, bladder or bowel sags into her vagina. It's common. About one in ten Australian women experience it.

How do I do pelvic floor exercises?

Sometimes women say that they don't know which muscles to contract. It's very easy to learn. Go to the toilet and urinate. During urination, attempt to stop the flow. Which muscles do you use? They are your pelvic floor muscles! It's okay to locate your pelvic floor muscles by stopping the flow of urine, but not wise to do this as a form of exercise. Theoretically, if done regularly, it could cause urine to back up, and cause kidney problems. These are the same muscles that you use when you attempt to prevent yourself from passing wind.

Sit propped up against a wall or bed head, and use a mirror and light to see your perineum (the area between your vagina and anus). When you do a pelvic

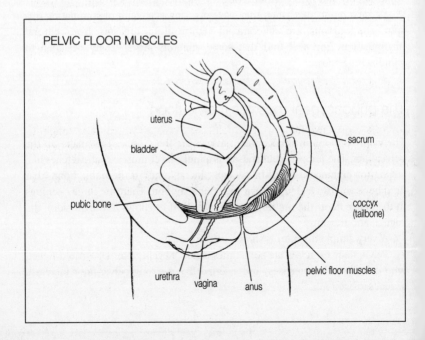

PELVIC FLOOR MUSCLES

uterus

bladder

sacrum

pubic bone

coccyx
(tailbone)

pelvic floor muscles

urethra   vagina   anus

floor contraction this area should lift upwards towards your abdomen. You should be able to feel and see a movement in the upward direction. You can also identify this movement by putting your finger on your perineum (the area between your vagina and anus). If you cannot see or feel a movement at first, you will be able to do so after exercising for a couple of months.

You can put your finger in your vagina and feel the strength of your muscles' contraction. You will be able to feel an increase in strength after you have been practising pelvic floor exercises for a month.

Who needs to do them?

I would advise all women to learn how to do Kegels and to do them regularly. The reason is that as we age many women experience urinary incontinence. Strengthening your pelvic floor muscles may not only improve your sex life, but will definitely enhance your quality of life as you age.

Learning your exercises

Exercise 1:
Contract your pelvic floor, hold for a count of three, and relax. It's the same movement as if you were trying to prevent yourself passing urine, wind or faeces. Squeeze as tightly as you can.

Repeat this five times. If you have a very weak pelvic floor, you may prefer to start your exercises when lying down so that there is no pressure on the pubococcygeus muscle from the weight above the muscle. As your muscles strengthen you can do the exercises sitting, lying, standing and while walking around.

Do a set of five contractions ten times per day.

Exercise 2:
Contract your pelvic floor muscles, hold for a count of three, then cough. If you are watching in the mirror you should not see a downward movement of your perineum.

Do this three times a day. Also do it any time you feel yourself about to cough or sneeze during the day.

Appendix 3:
Sexually Transmitted Infections

Sexually transmitted infections (previously called sexually transmitted diseases or STDs) are common. A woman who is well informed about them is equipped to make decisions about the kind of sexual activity she is prepared to be involved in.

Chlamydia

This common infection is often called 'the silent STI' because most people who have it do not have symptoms. It can be transmitted by touch and is not always easy to detect. In women it can cause pelvic inflammatory disease and decreased fertility. The organism may live in the urethra, cervix, rectum, throat and eyes. In women in may be detected by a urine test, or by a cervical swab. Cervical swabs may be collected when a woman has a Pap test, but unless you have asked the health worker to do a sexually transmitted infection screen when you have your Pap test, they may not do the extra chlamydia swab.

When symptoms are present they may include vaginal discharge or abnormal vaginal bleeding, pelvic pain, or pain while having sex. If chlamydia is detected, it can be treated by a course of antibiotics.

Genital herpes

Genital herpes is very common. It is estimated that among sexually active young people up to one-quarter may have this virus. It is equally prevalent among lesbian women and heterosexual women.[1]

Genital herpes is caused by the same type of virus that causes cold sores. Herpes can be transmitted by mouth to genital contact. If a cold sore on a lip or nose comes in to contact with the tender skin of the vulva or vagina the herpes virus can start a sore. If you do oral sex, a woman with a cold sore (or *any* sore) around her mouth is one of the most serious risks to lesbian sexual health. Vulva-to-vulva contact can transmit the virus. Fingers can also transmit the virus. If you finger a vulva which has herpes sores, and then touch a vulva, clitoris or anus (or any moist, tender skin) which was not previously infected, you can transmit the virus from one place to another.

In the past it was said that genital herpes was caused by the Herpes Simplex Virus Type II (HSV II) and cold sores on mouths were caused by Herpes Simplex Virus Type I (HSV I). We now know that YOU CAN GET BOTH TYPES IN BOTH PLACES. HSV I is often on the lips, and the genital symptoms may be less severe. HSVII tends to be on the genitals, and be more severe with more recurrences. But for practical purposes it makes no difference if you get it.

One way to prevent the transmission of herpes is not to have risky contact when a herpes sore is present. The virus is transmissible during the time when the sore is present and until the skin looks normal again (usually five to ten days).

It is now known that there is also a risk of transmission when no sore can be seen on the skin. This is called 'asymptomatic shedding'. It can happen when people do not even know they have got HSV because the symptoms have been so minor that they were overlooked. Most people who contract herpes get it from a partner who is asymptomatic.

Consider using safe sex practices to reduce the risk of herpes. If you are into casual sex with a number of partners, one of the best defences against herpes is to KEEP THE LIGHT ON! Have a look at your partner (this can be part of foreplay). Any sore or blistery lesion is a good reason not to touch that area or to use a barrier. However, skin on skin contact can transmit herpes and we don't know how to prevent this.

The symptoms of herpes vary. In a first attack there may be very painful blisters and sores. Sometimes, however, the blisters may be so small that they are not noticed. There may be a red sore area with small breaks in the skin. There may be tingling, itching, ulcers, difficulty in passing urine and flu-like symptoms. Recurrent attacks are usually milder than the first episode. There may be a feeling of being generally 'off-colour' and also genital itching or tingling. This is called the 'prodrome', and warns that an attack is on its way. Attacks may be very severe and debilitating, or they may be so mild that they are not noticed. Outbreaks become less frequent as time goes by.

Sometimes it is possible for a health worker to tell, just by looking, that the problem is herpes. However, to be absolutely sure, herpes is diagnosed by taking a swab from a sore or blister. Unfortunately, there are difficulties with the test, and it is possible to have herpes even if the test is negative.

The first episode of herpes, and severe recurrent attacks, may be treated by medications called 'anti-virals'. Treatment reduces the duration of the attack and may greatly reduce the number of outbreaks.

Occasionally, women will have one episode and then have no more. The first outbreak usually occurs two to twenty days after exposure to the virus. However, rarely, symptoms can appear for the first time months or even years after exposure.

Once the virus has caused an infection it remains living in the nerves that run from the spinal cord to the affected area. It lies dormant. This is the reason that many people have recurrent episodes. The virus reactivates and travels back down the nerve to the skin. Recurrent outbreaks may be so mild as to be no problem at all. For some women they are very distressing, and it seems that stress can sometimes bring on an attack. Some women notice that attacks occur when they are sunburnt or premenstrual. Others find that episodes happen when they have used drugs or had large amounts of alcohol. Sexual contact (either with another person or by masturbation) brings on attacks in some women.

People who have frequent, distressing recurrences may choose to have daily suppressive anti-viral medication, even when they are well. If you are having a hard time with herpes, you might choose to see your doctor to discuss this. It is worthwhile remembering that herpes often 'burns itself out'. However, there are a number of lifestyle, nutritional and herbal treatments for herpes (see 'Resources').

There are two ways to protect yourself from getting herpes: firstly, don't have sexual contact with anyone who has a cold sore, or any sort of a sore on their genitals – a sore is a herpes sore until proven otherwise. Secondly, because the virus can be transmitted when there are no sores present, it's wise to consider using dams and other barrier methods if you don't know whether or not your partner has had herpes.

Genital warts

Genital warts are caused by the human Papiloma virus (HPV). They are spread by contact. Direct touching of your partner's genital warts puts you at risk. This is true for both lesbian and heterosexual sex. Warts are common among both lesbian and heterosexual women.[2]

Warts may be flat and invisible to the naked eye. Or they may be visible as small lumps, which are sometimes cauliflower-shaped. They may be on the vulva, perineum and anus. Or they may be internal: inside the vagina or on the cervix. If they are internal, women are usually unaware that they are there unless they show up on a Pap test.

The wart virus may in time lead to the development of abnormal cells on the cervix. If they are untreated, over time these cells may change into cervical cancer. Advancing age and smoking increase the risk of cervical cancer. Risk also increases with the number of sexual partners that a woman has. It is lower for women who have not been sexually active, or who have had few partners, and higher for women who have had more partners. If a woman is HIV positive, her chance of getting cervical cancer also increases.

If you feel that you may have genital warts you should see your doctor or health professional for a physical examination and a Pap test. The Pap test is to work out whether the warts have started to make the cells of the cervix change.

Warts may be treated by applying podophylin paint. This is painted onto the warts by someone who can see what they are doing, usually a health professional. They can also be removed by freezing (cryotherapy), burning (diathermy), laser, or surgical removal. Warts are treated to reduce the area from which the virus may spread, and for cosmetic reasons. Removing the wart does not completely remove the virus. There is still a risk of them recurring, and of infecting someone else.

If you have genital warts, you should ensure that you have regular Pap tests. Your sexual partner(s) should have a sexual health check to determine whether or not she/they have warts too.

Gonorrhoea

This disease is caused by bacteria. It is transmitted by touch. Women often do not have any symptoms. If they do, the symptoms will occur two to seven days after contact. There may be pain on urinating or a vaginal discharge. It may not be diagnosed until a cervical swab is done. This infection is not common in the lesbian community but it does exist. There is no difference in the prevalence of this STI between straight women and women who have sex with women.[3]

There have been recent epidemics of gonorrhoea among gay men. Lesbians will sometimes sleep with gay men. Some will not have penetrative sex with a man, but may feel okay about giving a gay male friend a 'head job'.[4] These women may be at risk of gonorrhoea (and can pass it on to other women) because it may be transmitted by oral sex. You can get this infection in your mouth or throat. It is easily treated by a course of antibiotics, but if left untreated can lead to pelvic inflammatory disease and decreased fertility.

Hepatitis A, B & C

Hepatitis means 'inflamation of the liver'. There are a large number of different types. Many are caused by viruses. They are different viruses and they are identified by letters of the alphabet. Hepatitis can also be caused by a number of other organisms (including cytomegalovirus, Epstein-Barr virus and the herpes simplex viruses) and by toxins. Hepatitis A, B and C are different infections with differing symptoms and long-term effects, and dissimilar routes of transmission. These three are the ones with most impact on the lesbian community.

Hepatitis A

Hepatitis A is a virus that damages the liver. It is carried by bile into the gut and excreted in faeces. It is transmitted through contact with faeces, or by food or water that has been contaminated by faeces. The route is from the faeces of one person, through the mouth of the next. Eating contaminated oysters or shellfish can also transmit it. People who have anal sex are at risk from this infection.

The virus causes a debilitating illness, which can last several weeks. Most people recover completely in two to three months. A small number take much longer to recover. Very rarely, people die from acute hepatitis A.

Transmission is prevented by scrupulous cleanliness. It is possible to be vaccinated against this virus. If you ever have anal sex, it is worthwhile considering vaccination. There is now a combined HepA/HepB vaccine available.

Hepatitis B

Hepatitis B also causes liver inflammation and damage. The route of transmission is different. The virus is present in quantities that can cause infection in blood, vaginal secretions and saliva. Of all the life-threatening STIs, this one is the most contagious!

This virus may be transmitted by kissing, and by unprotected vaginal, anal or oral sex. It can be passed by sharing needles, syringes and drug-injecting equipment and also by childbirth (from an infected woman to her baby). Sharing toothbrushes, razors and other personal items that may be contaminated by bodily secretions may also result in transmission. Any form of blood-to-blood contact is highly risky. Contact with saliva is less risky.

When health workers talk about 'blood-to-blood contact', they mean that the blood of one person has passed into the bloodstream of another. This can happen if one person is injured and another person gets their blood into a cut or sore. It can also happen if menstrual blood gets into the cracks on a tongue or around teeth. Any way that the blood from one person gets through the broken skin of another may be sufficient to allow transmission.

Symptoms usually develop within three months after exposure and can range from a mild flu-like illness to jaundice (yellowing of the skin and the whites of the eyes) and serious illness. Most people who get hepatitis B recover and develop immunity. However, five to ten per cent of people may remain infectious for many years. They are called 'carriers', and can pass the infection on even though they are no longer sick themselves. A small percentage of people who contract hepatitis B may develop chronic active hepatitis and die from progressive liver damage or liver cancer.

The risk of transmission is reduced by safer sexual practices. This disease can be prevented by being vaccinated against the virus.

Hepatitis C

Some of the literature about hepatitis C states that it is not considered to be a sexually transmissible infection. I have included it in this appendix because it is a very common disease and because sexual transmission is not impossible. Between one and two Australians in every 200 carry this virus. Dr Fethers found that it was more common among women who have sex with women than among those who did not. Her survey was of an inner-city population which attended the Sydney Sexual Health Clinic. These women also reported more frequent injecting drug use than straight women.[5]

Transmission of hepatitis C is almost always through blood-to-blood contact (see above). The most common mode of transmission has been through sharing needles.

Sexual activity that does not involve blood-to-blood contact is said to be very low risk (but not no risk). It is thought that hepatitis C may be transmitted by sexual activity but only if the person with the virus has a very high viral load (for instance, in the initial stages of infection). It has been suggested that the risk of sexual transmission may be increased during the first six months of the disease. People who have hep C can have blood tests to determine their viral load.

When one partner is hepatitis C positive, it is important to ensure that sexual activity does not cause blood-to-blood contact. It is suggested that couples consider alternatives to oral sex, or use dams when the hep C positive partner is menstruating. Lots of lube to prevent skin damage is also important. It is also advised that rough sex which might damage mucus membranes or draw blood be avoided.

Up to twenty per cent of people who get hep C will be completely well again in two to six months. Sixty per cent will have a persistent infection lasting for years that may have effects ranging from mild (tiredness) to serious (profound malaise, nausea and abdominal pain). About twenty-five per cent have a long-term infection that leads to serious liver damage. Half of the twenty-five per cent with severe liver damage will die from liver failure or liver cancer. Hepatitis C is very variable in its effects but most people won't get really sick. When people do get sick, the disease usually takes a very long time to progress (ten to twenty years).

HIV/AIDS

The Human Immunodeficiency Virus (HIV) causes harm to the body's immune system. Acquired Immune Deficiency Syndrome (AIDS) is a condition that occurs as a late stage after infection by HIV. The virus may cause serious illness and death through damage to the immune system.

The HIV virus exists in body fluids. It can only cause infection when the body fluid of one person gets into the bloodstream of another. HIV is considered to be a 'fragile virus', that is, it dies very quickly when it is outside the human body. It cannot be passed on by sharing eating utensils. If the virus is swallowed, the acid in your stomach will kill it. It cannot gain entry to the human body through intact skin, only through cuts or abrasions, or by contact with mucus membranes (like the delicate lining of the rectum).

The HIV virus is found in different concentrations in different body fluids: blood (including menstrual blood), semen and breast milk contain concentrations of the virus that are known to transmit infection; vaginal fluid also contains the virus in lower concentrations, but still in sufficient quantity to transmit the virus.

Saliva may contain the virus, but not in sufficient quantities to permit transmission. The virus is not present in urine, faeces or vomit unless these substances also contain blood. There have been no cases recorded of infection by these routes.

Woman-to-woman oral sex is considered to be low risk (but not no risk). The risk is much higher if you have abrasions in your mouth or gum disease. Very few people could be sure that recent tooth-brushing had not left them with small breaks in the mucous membranes round their teeth.

Sexual activities that do not result in the blood or vaginal secretions getting into the bloodstream of another will not result in transmission of this virus. Unprotected vaginal and anal sex is considered to be high risk.

Mites

Pubic lice (sometimes called 'crabs') and scabies are tiny mites which cause itching. Pubic lice grip onto pubic hair. Scabies burrow under the skin to lay eggs. Both are transmitted by skin to skin contact and may also live in bed linen, towels or clothes. They can be identified by careful examination. Neither cause any serious complications and both can be cured by the appropriate lotions, creams or shampoo.

Pelvic inflamatory disease (PID)

The symptoms of PID include fever, abdominal pain, and pain on deep penetration during sexual activity. It can result in heavier, painful and irregular periods. There are various organisms that may lead to PID. These include chlamydia and gonorrhoea (see the sections on these organisms above). The bacteria causes infection of the uterus, fallopian tubes and surrounding organs. PID can be a serious illness requiring hospitalisation. If it is not treated it can cause infertility, and may increase the risk of ectopic pregnancies. Once it is detected, PID can be treated by antibiotics.

Syphilis

Syphilis is very rare among lesbian women, and is now uncommon in Australia's general population. I mention it only for completeness, as it is one of the better-known STIs. Symptoms in the early stage of the disease include painless sores. The symptoms of the second stage of the illness include a rash on the palms. It is transmitted by contact with the sores or the rash. If it is not treated, it causes serious illness and death. However, once diagnosed, it is effectively treated with antibiotics. It is detected by a blood test that should be part of every sexually transmitted infection screen.

Vaginal infections

Itch, burning vulva, and an increase in vaginal discharge, which may or may not have a disagreeable odor, are the usual symptoms of vaginal infection. They are more likely to occur if the vaginal environment is out of balance. This can be caused by emotional stress, chemical irritants (such as scents, douches, vulva deodorants, or perfumes impregnated in tampons, pads or toilet paper), high humidity (made worse by wearing synthetic underwear, especially during exercise). The vaginal environment changes before and after a woman's period. It may also change as a result of sex with a new partner, especially if the partner is a man (semen is an alkaline fluid which may increase vaginal ph for up to eight hours). There are several different types of vaginal infection:

Bacterial vaginosis

This is also known as 'BV'. It may be caused by the bacteria *Gardnerella vaginalis*, and by a variety or other organisms.

If the normal vaginal environment is altered, bacteria may grow in greater numbers than usual. BV causes a disagreeable smell and sometimes a thin grey vaginal discharge (which may be worse before menstruation and after sex). It can make oral sex unpleasant. However, fifty per cent of women who have BV do not have symptoms.

Health researchers are still in disagreement about whether or not BV can be sexually transmitted. However, Dr Fethers found that BV was significantly more prevalent among women who have sex with women. Research indicates that more frequent receptive oral sex could be associated with an increased risk of BV. The study found that eight to ten per cent of WSW had BV. Other researchers have found much higher rates of BV infection among lesbian women than among heterosexual women.[6] It is speculated that oral sex may be capable of transmitting these organisms.

BV is diagnosed by vaginal swab. A swab is like a sterile cotton bud, but has a longer handle. It is inserted into the vagina to absorb some of the discharge. This is then tested in a pathology laboratory.

This condition may be treated by a course of antibiotics.

Candidiasis or 'thrush'

This is a yeast infection caused by *Candida albicans*. It is particularly likely to occur after a woman has had a course of antibiotics (which as well as treating the bacteria they were intended for, may also kill off the vagina's normal 'healthy' bacteria). There are always yeast spores in a vagina, so when the 'good' bacteria are absent, the yeast flourishes. Some lesbian women find that particular lubes make them more prone to thrush.

This is not considered to be a sexually transmitted infection. However, heterosexual women who get repeated bouts sometimes find that when their partner is treated with an anti-fungal cream too, the problem settles. In theory, if a lesbian woman had thrush in her vagina, masturbated internally, then penetrated her partner she could pass the yeast on. However, whether or not you get candida also depends on your own immune system, and if you are a person who is prone to problems with thrush.

The discharge is thick and white or creamy yellow, and sometimes has a mild yeasty smell. The first sign of 'thrush' is usually itching. The vulva and vagina may become red and sore. The condition can often be diagnosed by a health worker doing a simple genital examination. If there is any uncertainty, the diagnosis can be confirmed by a vaginal swab.

Usually, anti-fungal creams or pessaries (tablets which are inserted into the vagina) will usually ease the condition quickly. Occasionally women get chronic candidiasis and may consider oral anti-fungal medication or natural therapies, including diets low in yeasts and sugars.

Women who have had the condition before often recognise it. Anti-fungal creams and pessaries are now sold by pharmacies over the counter (without the need for prescription). Many women start treatment as soon as the symptoms become a problem.

Trichomoniasis

This vaginal infection is caused by a parasite (*Trichomonas vaginalis*) that lives in the vagina of women and the urethra of men. It can be transmitted by contact, including vulva-to-vulva contact. Many women do not notice any symptoms. Some experience a yellow discharge and a vaginal odour. The parasite is easily diagnosed by vaginal swab. It causes no serious complications and is cured by a single dose of an antibiotic.

What to do if you think you might have an STI

See your doctor or health worker. Many sexually transmitted infections can be eradicated with antibiotics. There are medications that can assist, even when there is no 'cure'. Don't let embarrassment or fear put your health at risk. Find a health practitioner you can relate to and have a check-up!

Glossary

BABY BUTCH A younger lesbian exploring butch roles.

BISEXUAL A person who is sexually active with people of both genders or attracted to people of both genders.

BDSM This is one of the currently used abbreviations for 'bondage and discipline' or 'bondage and dominance' and 'sadism and masochism.' For more information, see 'Resources'.

BOTTOM In BDSM, a submissive participant.

BUTCH From the 1920s through to the early 1970s, many lesbians felt that they had to identify as either 'butch' or 'femme'. Often, women modelled their relationships with each other on the heterosexual model. One partner took the masculine role and the other took the feminine role. In the 1970s, lesbian feminist theory asserted that lesbian relationships were about women loving women. All the attributes of women, including both the soft and nurturing and the assertive and virile aspects, could live and be treasured in the same female human. It became 'unfashionable' to identify in this way. Nevertheless, many women who had always seen themselves as butch held to their identification. In contemporary Australian lesbian culture, some women enjoy exploring the strong, virile, active, assertive parts of their personalities. They may identify as butch. However, it is now seen as much more a fluid part of a continuum than 'either/or'. In very recent years there has been a resurgence of interest in butch/femme role dynamics.

CAMP Campaign Against Moral Persecution, a civil liberties group formed to fight for gay rights in 1970. 'Camp' was also used by gay men and lesbian women as a term to identify themselves.

CUNT Female genitals. This word is used proudly by lesbian feminists to describe the region which includes the vagina and the vulva. In other contexts it has been used as a term of contempt to describe women, particularly when they are seen as sexual objects.

CUNNILINGUS Oral stimulation of the female genitals. The word comes from the Latin words *cunnus* for vulva and *lingere* 'to lick'. It is commonly called 'going down on' and 'eating' or 'oral sex'. There is no law against oral sex in Australia or England. However, in some states in the United States it is a criminal offence.

DILDO An object designed to penetrate a vagina or anus for sexual pleasure.

DRAG KING A woman who likes dressing as a man. She will often do this when going out to pubs, shows and parties, but will retain her usual manner of dress at other times. She may have a male character with a male name that she takes on, just for the evening. Other women live their drag king character more frequently, but still identify as female, and lesbian, dyke, queer or bi-sexual.

DYKE This word was originally a derogatory word, slung at lesbians (as in 'You're a fuckin' dyke'). In the early 1970s, lesbian feminists chose to reclaim the word, answering proudly 'Yes, I'm a dyke'. For over twenty years, some lesbians have been extremely comfortable with the word, using it to dispel their own internal homophobia by claiming it as their own. In the 1990s many lesbians identify their sexual orientation, stating 'I'm a dyke' without a second thought. Some lesbians, however, remain uncomfortable with the term.

FAECES 'Waste matter discharged from bowels',[1] also called poo, pooh, shit, turds, crap, etc.

FEMME This comes from the French word which means 'woman'. It refers to women who take the feminine roles in lesbian relationships. In times gone by, lesbians felt that they had to identify as either 'butch' or 'femme'. Since the 1970s many lesbians have seen themselves as 'women loving women' rather than adopting butch or femme roles. An acceptance of gender fluidity has more recently led to an upsurge in the number of women affecting a femme lesbian identity. (See also 'butch' and 'lipstick lesbian'.)

FELLATIO Sucking or licking a penis.

FINGER FUCKING, FINGERING See p. 50.

FISTING See p.50.

FROTTAGE Another word for Tribadism. See below and also p. 45.

GAY A term used by homosexual women and men to describe themselves and define their sexual orientation. It was probably first used in this way in the 1930s and has been in wide use since the 1960s.[2] Women who do not like the word 'lesbian' often use it to describe themselves. In recent times it has been used more by gay men. Hence we have the 'Gay and Lesbian Mardi Gras'. The Australian Gay Medical Association is an association for men. However, many women continue to name themselves as gay. There is a perception held by some feminist lesbians that women who call themselves 'gay' are choosing to be less political than women who term themselves 'lesbian' or 'dyke'.

GLBT Gay, Lesbian, Bi-sexual, Transgender.

GOLDEN SHOWERS See 'water sports'.

HEAD JOB Mouth to penis sex. Also called fellatio. Some women also use this term for oral sex with women (cunnilingus).

HERSTORY In her book *Gyn/Ecology*,[3] Mary Daly points out that the way we use language structures our thinking. Feminists use 'herstory' as a way of reminding their listeners that most of our records have been written by men (and are from their perspective). The important achievements of women have often been unrecorded. Women are now writing chronicles that document our stories.

HETEROSEXUAL A person who is attracted to and has sex with a person of the opposite sex.

HETEROSEXUAL PRIVILEGE see p. 144

HOMOSEXUAL This term was coined in 1869 by Dr Karol Maria Benket. In the 1890s, it was adopted by Havelock Ellis, an English sexologist.[4] It continues to be the established term favoured by the medical profession and most other professionals. It is less commonly used for self-description. It has been argued that to use this term as a description of one's own identity buys into medical pathologising of same-sex sexual orientation.[5]

INCONTINENCE Releasing urine or faeces without intending to. Usually if women talk about incontinence they mean urinary incontinence. It's very common. At least one in three women who have had a baby will have some urinary incontinence.

INVERT A term used from 1864 to the mid-1900s referring to homosexual people. In 1864 Karl Ulrichs published a pamphlet about a 'third sex' – women trapped in men's bodies. He termed this 'inversion', and the trapped people were referred to as 'inverts'.

LABRYS The ancient double-bladed axe, said in mythology to have been wielded by the 'Amazons', who defended the Goddess's shrine at Delphi. In modern times, lesbians have adopted the symbol. Represented in jewellery or art, it is often used as a means of identifying another lesbian. At one time, lesbian separatists saw it as their own particular symbol.

LEATHER DYKE A lesbian for whom part of her identity includes wearing leather. She may or may not see herself as butch. She may or may not be interested or involved in BDSM. She may or may not be interested in motorbikes.

LESBIAN A woman who is sexually attracted to women. A female homosexual. Large numbers of lesbians are comfortable with this term for themselves. Some women do not like the word and prefer to call themselves 'gay'.

LESBIAN FEMINIST A lesbian with feminist politics.

LESBIAN SEPARATIST A lesbian who chooses not to associate with men.

LESBIAN WOMAN It has been suggested that the phrase 'lesbian woman' repeats the same concept. By definition, a lesbian is a woman. Many feminist thinkers, however, prefer this term to 'lesbian', stating that it is not helpful to define human beings by words that classify on the basis of sexual orientation. They argue that each lesbian woman is much more than her sexual orientation. She may be a sister, daughter, mother, writer, doctor, cook, cleaner, lawyer, animal lover, artist, musician or poet as well. Each lesbian woman is a complex person. I therefore use the terms 'lesbian' and 'lesbian woman' interchangeably to remind readers of our multiple facets.

LGBT Commonly used abbreviation for Lesbian, Gay, Bi-sexual and Transgender

LIBIDO Sexual desire or drive.

LIPSTICK LESBIAN A lesbian who likes to wear lipstick, 'feminine' clothes etc. She may or may not see herself as 'femme'.

MONS, MONS PUBIS The rounded fleshy mound over a woman's pubic bone. Also known as the 'pubic mound'. Sometimes known as 'the mound of Venus'.

NON-SCENE A lesbian who is not involved in the scene. (See 'scene'). Lesbians who are 'non-scene' are often involved in family life, personal interests, friendships, entertaining at home, sport and similar activities.

PASSING To pass as straight. Not to be known as lesbian. Also, this word is used by women who have chosen to pass as men and live their lives in male roles.

ORAL SEX See 'cunnilingus' above and p. 46.

QUEER Homosexual, gay, lesbian, bisexual, transgender, SMBD, fetishist, whatever. Any sexual identity that is not heterosexual. Queer was historically used as a term of abuse for homosexuals. From 1910 gay men have used the word to describe themselves. However, since the 1990s the word 'queer' has taken on new meanings. It has been reclaimed and mobilised by non-heterosexuals. It is non-specific and inclusive. There is no agreement on the exact definition of 'queer'.[6]

RIMMING Licking or sucking around the anus.

SCAT Sex play with faeces.

SCENE Refers to places to meet (pubs and clubs), activities (dancing, drugs, alcohol), events (Mardi Gras, lesbian cultural festivals), interests (lesbian services, campaigns for social justice) and personality style (young, cool, very 'out', uninhibited sexuality). 'Scene' is also used by SM dykes to describe a fantasy scenario that is being played out.

SEPARATIST See 'lesbian separatist'.

SM Sadomasochism. See p. 56.

STD Sexually transmitted disease. See also 'STI'.

STI Sexually transmitted infection. As not all sexually transmitted infections actually cause disease, this is the term currently preferred by many Australian sexual health workers.

STONE BUTCH '...a (butch) lesbian who gives her femme lover pleasure but will not allow the femme to touch her sexually, penetrate or bring her to orgasm'.[7]

STRAIGHT Heterosexual. Also, sometimes used to refer to the state of not being under the influence of alcohol or drugs.

STRESS INCONTINENCE Urinary incontinence caused by a sudden increase in intra-abdominal pressure. Often from unexpectedly sneezing, lifting or laughing.

TOP In BDSM, a dominant participant.

TRANSGENDER/ TRANSGENDER PERSON A person who was born with the anatomical characteristics of one gender, but who has the strong desire to adopt the physical characteristics and role of the other gender, or who believes that they are of the other gender. The person may or may not have had surgical treatment to alter the external sexual features so that they resemble those of the opposite sex. They may also take prescribed hormones to aid the transformation. A person who lives (or wants to live) as a person of the other gender.

TRANSVESTITE A person who dresses in the clothes of the opposite sex. The person may or may not see themselves as transsexual or transgender. History records many stories of lesbian women who were transvestite and who chose to live their lives as men. Many may have seen themselves as transgender people. Lesbian women may like to adopt male roles for short or long periods. They may choose to wear male clothes for this purpose. At times lesbian fashion has dictated male attire. Women sometimes like to wear male clothes for the freedom it gives, or the way it makes them feel, while continuing to identify as female.

TRANSSEXUAL See 'Transgender'.

TRIBADISM See p. 45.

VANILLA LESBIAN Lesbian who likes vanilla lesbian sex. (See below.)

VANILLA SEX A term used to describe lesbian sexual practice that does not include SM, BD, Sub/dom, etc.[8] Originally coined by some lesbians as a derogatory term to describe an idea of lesbian sex which seemed limited and proscriptive. In contemporary use it has been reclaimed with a positive frame.

VULVA A woman's external genitals. Includes the pubic mound (mons pubis), the inner and outer lips of the vagina (labia majoria and minora), the clitoris and the vaginal opening.

WATER SPORTS Sexual activity that involves playing with urine.

WSW Women who have sex with women. This is a description of behaviour, used to define a group of women. It does not rely on their internal perception of themselves, but on what they do. It is used by researchers, and also by some women to identify themselves.

WOMEN-BORN-WOMEN There are male to female transgender people who identify as lesbian. In an effort to distinguish between lesbians who started life as women and those who started life as men, some lesbians (and some lesbian organisations) refer to 'women-born-women'.

Resources

This selection of resources should be regarded as a sample of what is available rather than an exhaustive list. There are many more entries that could be included. If you know of a resource that you would like to see on this list, please email me: carolbooth@gay.com. I will then include it in the next edition. If you are associated with an organisation that has changed its contact details, please also let me know. Every effort has been made to check that this list is accurate. If you find an inaccuracy, please email me.

I would like to express my thanks to the wonderful women of the Feminist Bookshop and the staff of the Darlinghurst Bookshop for their generous and uncomplaining help.

- Accoutrements
- Addiction
- BDSM
- Bisexuality
- Bookshops
- Contacts
- Counselling
- Coming Out
- Discrimination
- Feeling Good About Your Body
- Festivals
- Health
- Herpes
- Homophobia
- Immigration
- Intersex and Androgynous People
- Lesbians and the Law
- Lesbian Lives
- Lesbian Sex
- Lesbian Women With Disabilities
- Making Babies and Parenting
- Masturbation
- Media
- Menopause
- Older Lesbians
- Parents of Lesbians
- Politics
- Reference and Research
- Relationship Issues
- Search Engines and Email Lists
- Self-Esteem
- Sex Addiction
- Sexual Assault
- Sex and Spirituality
- Spirituality Generally
- Transgender Issues
- Violence and Physical Abuse
- Young Lesbians

Accoutrements

Dams may be purchased from any of the sex shops listed here. They may also be available free at some dance parties, or for a moderate price from the various AIDS Councils (see below), family planning organisations, many women's health centres, and some pharmacies. Website: kiaorapacific.com.au.

Downunder Toys PO Box 7356, Melbourne, Vic 3004. Sex toys – made by women for women. Tel/fax: 03 9827 9744.
Email: downundertoys@hotmail.com. Website: www.downundertoys.com.au.

Lesbian-friendly sex shops
The Toolshed Newtown Tel: 02 9565 1599. Darlinghurst Tel: 02 9332 2792.
The Pleasure Spot PO Box 213, Woollahra, NSW 2025. Tel: 02 9361 0433.
Fax: 02 9331 6120. Email: pleaspot@ozemail.com.au. Website:
www.pleasurespot.net.

Online Products
LexySmart.com Australia's only online shop for lesbian and bisexual women. Wide range of adult products, discreet packaging.

Addiction

Arcadia House, Canberra Gay & Lesbian educated drug and alcohol detox. Does take same-sex couples. Tel: 02 6253 3055.
GLIDUP (Gay and Lesbian Injecting Drug Use Project) Tel: 02 9206 2096.
WIREDD (Women's Information, Resources and Education on Drugs and Dependency) Canberra Tel: 02 6248 8600.

Groups
Alcoholics Anonymous, Narcotics Anonymous and a large number of other organisations that will assist with drug and alcohol addiction may be found in the yellow pages of the phone book.

Books
Drescher, Jack, Guss, Jeffrey, 2000, *Addictions in the Gay and Lesbian Community*, Haworth Press.
Melody, Pia and Wells, Andrea, 1989, *Facing Co-Dependence*, HarperCollins.
Melody, Pia and Wells, Andrea, 1989, *Breaking Free*, HarperCollins. (Note: this is the workbook for *Facing Co-Dependence*.)

BDSM

Contacts
See 'Media' below. Numerous contacts may be found in the gay newspapers of the various states.

Books
ACON, 2000, *Spank Elektric: Dyke SM Revealed*, ACON.

Brame, Gloria, 2001, *Come Hither: A Common Sense Guide to Kinky Sex*, Fusion Press.

Califa, Pat, *The Lesbian S/M Safety Manual*, Alyson Publication.

Califa, Pat, 1997, *Bitch Goddess: The Spiritual Path of the Dominant Woman*, Greenery Press.

Devon, Molly and Miller, Phillip, 1995, *Screw The Roses, Send Me the Thorns*, Mystic Rose Books.

Green, Lady (ed.) with Jaymes Easton, 1998, *Kinky Craft – 99 Do It Yourself SM Toys for the Kinky Handyperson*, Greenery Press.

Easton, Dossie and Liszt, Catherine A., 1998, *The Topping Book*, Greenery Press.

Easton, Dossie and Liszt, Catherine A., 1998, *The Bottoming Book*, Greenery Press.

Easton, Dossie and Liszt, Catherine A., 2000, *When Someone You Love Is Kinky*, Greenery Press.

Mistress Lorelei, 2000, *The Mistress Manual: The Good Girl's Guide To Female Dominance*, Greenery Press.

Wiseman, Jay, 1996, *SM 101*, Greenery Press.

Wiseman, Jay, 2000, *Erotic Bondage Handbook*, Greenery Press.

Warren, John, 2000, *The Loving Dominant*, Greenery Press.

Websites
Greenery Press www.greenerypress.com
BDSM index www.sexuality.org/bdsm.html
ALT sex www.altsex.org

Bisexuality

Contacts
Albury Wodonga Bisexual Group Email: borderbisexuals@icqmail.com.
Australian Bisexual Network Tel: 07 3857 2500, or if phoning from outside Brisbane, 1800 653 223. Email: ausbinet@rainbow.net.au.
Website: http://www.rainbow.net.au/ausbinet/.
Sydney Bisexual Network Tel: 02 9565 4281.

Websites

Australian Bisexual Network http://www.rainbow.net.au/~ausbinet/
Sydney Bisexual Network http://sbn.bi.org/
Sydney BiFem Social Group http://sydneybifem.freeservers.com/index.html
Sydney Bi and Poly Group
    http://sydneyinteractive.virtualave.net/html/index.html

Books

Garber, M.B., 1996, *Vice Versa: Bisexuality and the Eroticism of Everyday Life*,
    Simon & Schuster.
Hutchins, Loranie, Kaahumanu, 1991, *Bi any other name. Bisexual people
    speak out*, Alyson Books.
Klein, Fritz, MD, 1993, *The Bisexual Option*, 2nd ed., Harrington Park Press.
Rose, Sharon, Stevens, Cris, et al., 1998, *Bisexual Horizons Politics Histories
    Lives*, Lawrence & Wisheart.
Storr, Merl, 1999, *Bisexuality: A Critical Reader*, Routledge.

Bookshops

Why, you may wonder, would I list bookshops? These bookshops are not
ordinary bookshops. They will be able to provide you with lots of fantastic
lesbian resources! Many take phone orders, and will advise about books to
suit your particular needs.

NSW

Feminist Bookshop Shop 9, Orange Grove Plaza, Balmain Road, Lilyfield,
NSW 2020. Tel: 02 9810 2666. Fax: 02 9818 5745. The '...oldest, wisest,
most beautiful women's bookshop...' in Australia! Provides advice on
resources and offers an Australia-wide postal service.

The Darlinghurst Bookshop 207 Oxford Street, Darlinghurst, NSW 2010.
Tel: 02 9331 1103. Email: info@thebookshop.com.au. Gay Bookshop with
lots of BDSM resources.

QLD

Women's Bookshop 15 Gladstone Road, Highgate Hill, Qld 4101.
Tel: 07 3844 6650. Email: wimbooks@ribbon.net.au.
Website: www.thewomensbookshop.com.au.

VIC

Hares & Hyenas 135 Commercial Rd, South Yarra, Vic 3141. Tel: 03 9824
0110.

WA

Arcane Bookshop 212 William Street, Northbridge, WA 6000.
Tel: 08 93285073. Fax: 08 9228 0410. Email: arcbooks@highway1.com.au.

NZ
Women's Bookshop 105 Ponsonby Rd, Auckland. Tel: 64 376 4399.
Website: www.womensbookshop.co.nz.

Contacts

Special interest groups and social groups
aLBa (Auckland Lesbian Business Association) Website: cloud9@pl.net.
ALSO Foundation 35 Cato St, Prahran, Vic 3181. Tel: 03 9510 5569 for
GLBT resource directory. Email: also@also.org.au. Website: www.also.org.au.
Anbar South Asian Gay & Lesbian social group in Melbourne (speak to
Sudath), picnics, gatherings at people's homes, film nights. Tel: 03 9481 1424.
Australian Lesbian Medical Association (ALMA) National Australian
Association of Lesbian Doctors. PO Box 4042, Norwood South, SA 5067.
Website: www.almas.net.au.
Clover Women's Club The very first Australian lesbian social group.
(Sydney) Tel: Jan 02 9560 1154.
Dykes on Bikes Sydney: Tel: Janet 0404 265 806, Melbourne: Email:
dob@yahoo.com.au. Website: www.aardvark.net.au/~dobvic.
Brisbane: PO Box 1642, Fortitude Valley, Qld 4006.
JJ's Dance School Jan Blanch, Annandale (NSW). Tel: 02 9363 4735.
Juicy Fruit Lesbian social group. Open-age group. Social Sporting and
cultural alternatives to 'the scene'. Tel: Gaye 0414 285951. Email:
raindolph@hotmail.com..
Hobart Women's Health Centre This women's health centre employs a
lesbian health worker. Tel: 03 6231 3212.
Irish Lesbian and Gay Group PO Box 56, Alexandria, NSW 1435.
Tel: 02 9516 2174.
Lemons With A Twist Social evening presented regularly by the Gay and
Lesbian Business Association. Tel: 0438 196 998 (NSW), 03 9735 3630 (Vic).
Lesbian and Gay Pride WA Inc PO Box 30 North Perth, WA 6906.
Tel: 08 9227 1767. Email: pride@pridewa.asn.au.
Website: www.pridewa.asn.au.
Lesbian Support Group (Newcastle, NSW) Working Women's Centre.
Tel: 02 4968 2511.
Lesbian Teachers Group Ann Tel: 0401 011 929.
Website: http://lesbianteachers.tripod.com.
Les Singles Social group to find new friends. Tel: Linda 02 9630 6738 or
0415 805 840.
Literary Lesbians Reading group for under 30s. Tel: Alisa 02 9590 4542.
Melbourne Marching Girls PO Box 1095 North Fitzroy, Vic 3068.

Professional Women's Club Lesbians in professional or business roles.
Tel: 02 9518 9150. Email: profwomen@bigpond.com.
Pride Centre 281 Karangahape Rd, Auckland City. Tel: 64 9 302 590.
Fax: 0064 9 303 204. Email: pride@xtra.co.nz.
Rainbow Women's Network Professional women's network. PO Box 413,
Zillmere, Brisbane, Qld 4034. Tel: 07 3266 5284. Email: rwn@ribbon.net.au.
Sydney Asian Lesbians PO Box 817, Newtown, NSW 2042. Email:
asianlez@excite.com.au.
Sydney Gay and Lesbian Choir PO Box 649, Darlinghurst, NSW 1300.
Tel: 02 9360 7439. Fax: 02 9360 7439. Email: choir@sglc.org.
Website: www.sglc.org.
Sydney Gay and Lesbian Business Association PO Box 394, Darlinghurst,
NSW 1300. Tel: 02 9552 2000. Website: http//:www.gaybusiness.com.au.
Sydney Lesbian and Gay Community Centre Inc (Sydney Pride).
PO Box 7, Darlinghurst, NSW 1300. Tel: 02 9331 1333. Fax: 02 9331 1199.
Email: mail@pridecentre.com.au. Website: www.pridecentre.com.au.
Community centre: 26 Hutchinson Street, Surry Hills, NSW 2010. The
goal of the organisation is to facilitate gay and lesbian groups by providing
space and time.
The Women's Library 8–10 Brown St, Newtown, NSW 2042.
PO Box 271, Newtown, NSW 2042. Tel: 02 9557 7060.
Fax: 02 9557 5720.
WIRE (Women's Information Referral Exchange) Information and
support. Drop-in centre: 247 Flinders Lane, Melbourne, Vic 3000.
Tel: 1300 134 130. Email: wire@wire.org.au.
Women With Disabilities Australia (WWDA) PO Box 605, Rosny Park,
Tas 7018. Tel: 03 6244 8288, 03 6253 5104. Fax: 03 6244 8255.
Email: wwda@ozemail.com.au. Website: http://www.wwda.org.au.

Contact people in social groups change frequently. These details are correct at
the time of going to press. However, you are encouraged to check the lesbian
media for current details if you should find these outdated. (See below.) In
addition to the groups listed above, a large number of varied social and
sporting groups advertise in the lesbian magazines of the various states.

Regional social groups
In every state there are regional and local lesbian and gay social groups. The
lesbian newsletters and magazines listed under 'Media' provide contact
details. 'Lesbian Network' lists regional contacts all over Australia. You could
consider subscribing, or obtain a copy from the bookshop nearest you. The
Feminist Bookshop will take telephone orders and post nationwide, as will
many of the other bookshops.

Another way to make contact with a regional social group is to contact the closest AIDS Council. Every capital city in Australia, and many larger country towns, have an AIDS Council. Ring directory enquiries or look up the white pages to find out where the nearest one to you is. Many of the AIDS Councils are now very inclusive of lesbian women. Ask if there is a lesbian health worker. If there is, speak to her. If not, explain that you would like to make contact with the local lesbian and gay community. Even if it is not, strictly speaking, their job, many workers employed at the various AIDS Councils are very helpful and will give you contact numbers as a starting point.

Also, consider purchasing Ned Drinnan's *The Rough Guide to Gay and Lesbian Australia*, 2001, Penguin Australia, Ringwood, Victoria. (Email: maila@roughguides.com.auk. Website: www.oz.dreadedned.com.) This is currently available at most bookshops and large newsagents.

Counselling

If you are in need of urgent counselling please call Lifeline on 13 11 14. Or the Kids Help Line on 1800 55 1800.

AIDS Councils
While the main role of AIDS Councils is to assist people with HIV/AIDS, many offer groups or workshops aimed to present information about living as a gay person. Some of the Aids Counsel have a lesbian health worker. Many offer counselling to lesbian women.

ACT
AIDS Action Council Westlund House, 16 Gordon St, Acton, ACT 2601. Tel: 02 6257 2855. Fax: 02 6257 4838. Email: aidsaction@aidsaction.org.au.

NSW
ACON Western Sydney PO Box 350, Darlinghurst, NSW 1300.
Tel: 02 9206 2000. Fax: 02 98912088. TTY: 02 9283 2088.
Email: Aconwest@acon.org.au. Website: http://www.acon.org.au.
AIDS Council of NSW 9 Commonwealth St, Darlinghurst, NSW 2010.
Tel: 02 9206 2000. Rural callers: 1800 063 060. Fax: 02 9206 2002.
Website: http://www.rainbow.net.au/~acon/acon@acon.org.au.

NT
Northern Territory AIDS Council 46 Woods St, Darwin, NT 0800.
Tel: 08 8941 1711. Fax: 08 8941 2590. Email: info@ntac.org.au.

QLD
Queensland AIDS Council 32 Teel St, South Brisbane, Qld 4101.
Tel: 07 3017 1777. Freecall: 1800 177 434. Fax: 07 3844 4260.
Email: info@quac.org.au.
SA
AIDS Council of SA PO Box 907, Kent Town, SA 5071. Tel: 08 8362
1611 or 1800 888 559. Fax: 08 8363 1046. Email:
information@aidscouncil.org.au. Website: http://www.aidscouncil.org.au.
TAS
**TasCAHRD (Tasmanian Council of Aids, Hepatitis and Related
Diseases)** GPO Box 595, Hobart, Tas 7001. Tel: 03 6234 1242 or 1800 633
900. Email: mail@ tascahrd.org.au. Website: www.tascahrd.org.au.
VIC
Victorian AIDS Council 6 Claremont St, South Yarra, Vic 3141. Tel: 03
9865 6700. Fax: 03 9826 2700. Email: finhr@vicaids.asn.au.
WA
West Australian AIDS Council 664 Murray St, West Perth, WA 6005.
Tel: 08 9482 0000.

Lesbian and gay counselling services
ACT
Gay Information and Support Service Information Line ACT GPO Box
229, Canberra, ACT 2061. Tel: 02 6247 2726. Fax: 02 6257 4838.
Lesbian Line GPO Box 1645, Canberra, ACT 2601. Tel: 0402 168 336.
NSW
Gay and Lesbian Counselling Service 197 Albion Street (PO Box 334),
Darlinghurst, NSW 2010. Tel: 02 9207 2800 or 1800 184 527 (4 pm to
midnight). Fax: 02 9207 2828.
Email: glcs@bigpond.com. Website: www.glcsnsw.org.au.
Newcastle Gay and Lesbian Information and Support Service
Tel: 02 4929 6733 or 1800 184 527
QLD
Gay and Lesbian Welfare Association PO Box 1078, Fortitude Valley, Qld
4006.
Lesbianline 07 3891 7388. Toll free for rural areas: 1800 249 377. Gayline:
07 3891 7377. Email: glwa@queer.org.au. Website: http://glwa.queer.org.au.
SA
Gay and Lesbian Counselling Service of SA PO Box 2011, Kent Town, SA
5071. Tel: 08 8362 3223. Toll free for rural areas: 1800 182 233. Fax: 08
8363 1048. Website: www.glcssa.org.au.
Bfriend Department of Human Services Gay and Lesbian Support Service.
Tel: 08 8202 5192.

TAS
Gayline Tasmania Tel: 03 6234 8179. AIDS Info: 1800 005 900.
VIC
Gay and Lesbian Switchboard Tel: 03 9510 5488, 03 9510 1846.
Toll free for rural areas: 1800 631493.
Email: glswitch@vicnet.net.au http:www.vicnet.net.au/~glswitch.
WA
Gay and Lesbian Community Services of WA GPO Box 8146, Perth WA
6001. Tel: 08 9420 7201, 1800 184 527. Fax: 08 9223 1184. The line is
open 7.30–10 pm Monday to Friday. It has a special service for young
people, open Tuesdays 1–4 pm. The women's counsellor is available on
Wednesdays, 7.30–10 pm. (Crisis Care Line: 08 9223 1111, 1800 199 008,
TTY 9325 1232.)
**If you are in the Northern Territory, please consider calling South
Australia or Western Australia.**
New Zealand
Lesbianline Tel: 64 9 303 3584.
LESO Lesbian Education and Support Organisation PO Box 3833,
Auckland. Tel: 64 9 528 5119.

Other sources of counselling
Choosing a counsellor is something that should always be done carefully.
Counsellors who may (or may not) be familiar with lesbian issues can
sometimes be found at Women's Health Centres. *Lesbians on the Loose* and
some of the other lesbian magazines listed under 'Media' contain advertising
by lesbian and lesbian-friendly counsellors. The gay and lesbian telephone
advice service that serves your state will be able to suggest counselling
options.
Quest for Life Centre Petrea King and Wendie Batho run residential
workshops for women living with life-threatening illness or dealing with grief,
loss or trauma. PO Box 190, Bundanoon, NSW 2578. Tel: 02 4883 6599.
Email: petrea@questforlife.com.au. Website: http://www.questforlife.com.au.
HeartCentre Georgia Carr and Susan MacFarlane offer counselling and
residential workshops (personal and spiritual growth). They have been
working together in this field since 1980. Inspiration Place, Berrilee, NSW
2159. Tel: 02 9655 1055. Email: heartc@zeta.org.au.
Website: heartcentre.com.au.
Sophia College of Counselling Holistic counselling and training for
counsellors. Bunbury, WA 6230. Tel: 08 9731 5022, 08 9752 4569.
Email: sophia.college@bigpond.com.
See also 'Physical & Sexual Abuse' and 'Sexual Assault' below.

Books

Bettinger, Michael, 2001, *It's Your Hour: A Guide to Queer Affirmative Psychotherapy*, Alyson Books.

Black, Claudia, 1992, *Double Duty: Raised in an Alcoholic/Dysfunctional Family and Gay/Lesbian*, Mac Publishing.

Ernst, Sheila, and Goodison, Lucy, 1981, *In Our Own Hands: A Book of Self-Help Therapy*, The Woman's Press, London.

Waugh, Riggin, 2000, *Dykes with Baggage: The Lighter Side of Lesbians in Therapy*, Alyson Books.

Coming out

Books

Abbot, Deborah and Farmer, Ellen, 1995, *From Wedded Wife to Lesbian Life*, The Crossing Press.

Bono, Chastity, 1999, *Family Outing*, Bantam Publications.

Borhek, Mary, 1993, *Coming Out to Parents,* The Pilgrim Press.

Jensen, Karol, 1999, *Lesbian Epiphanies,* Harrington Park Press.

Shale, Erin, 1997, *Inside Out,* Bookman Publications.

Websites

Coming Out http://cust.idl.com.au//unsane/

The coming out of a lesbian mother: print it out and give it to your mum! http:/www.angelfire.com/co/lesmom/index/htm

A really useful gay man's coming out story: http:/www.angelfire.com/ga/outcome/

Discrimination

New South Wales, the Northern Territory, Queensland, South Australia and Victoria all have legislation protecting lesbian and gay people from discrimination as a result of their sexual orientation.

ACT Human Rights Office. GPO Box 158, Canberra ACT 2601. Tel: 02 6207 0576. TTY: 02 6207 0525. Email: humanrights@act.gov.au. Website: http://www.hro.act.gov.au.

NSW NSW Anti-Discrimination Board. PO Box A2122, Sydney South, NSW 1234. Tel: 02 9268 5555 or 1800 670 812. TTY: 02 9268 5522. Websites: http: www.lawlink.nsw.gov.au/adb, http: www.lawlink.nsw.gov.au/adb.nsf/pages/lesbian.

NT Northern Territory Anti-Discrimination Commission. Locked Mail Bag 22, GPO, Darwin, NT 0801. Tel and TTY: 08 8981 3813. Freecall: 1800 813 846. Fax: 08 8981 3812. Email: Administration.ADC@nt.gov.au.
QLD Queensland Anti-Discrimination Commission. PO Box 2122, Milton, Qld 4064. Tel: 1300 130 670. Website: http://www.adcq.qld.gov.au.
SA South Australia. Equal Opportunity Commission. GPO Box 464, Adelaide, SA 5001. Freecall: 1800 188 163. Email: eoc@agd.sa.gov.au. Website: http://www.eoc.sa.gov.au/public/sexuality.html.
TAS Office of the Anti-Discrimination Commissioner, GPO Box 197, Hobart, Tas 7001. Tel: 03 6234 3599. Freecall: 1800 001 222.
VIC Equal Opportunity Commission. Level 3/380 Lonsdale Street. Melbourne, Vic 3000. Tel: 03 9281 7111. TTY: 03 9281 7110. Freecall: 1800 134 142. Email: eoc@vicnet.net.au. Website: http://www.eoc.vic.gov.au.
WA Western Australia does not have legislation protecting gay and lesbian people from discrimination. They do, however, have an Equal Opportuntiy Commission. Tel: 08 9216 3900.

Feeling good about your body

Books
Baker, Jo Anne, 1998, *Self-Sexual Healing; Finding Pleasure Within*, Allen & Unwin, Sydney. (Jo Anne Baker, runs 'The Pleasure Spot' – see below.)
Dodson, Betty, 1996, *Sex For One: The Joy of Self-Loving*, Three Rivers Press, New York.
Henderson, Julie, 1986, *The Lover Within: Opening to Energy in Sexual Practice*, Station Hill Press, New York.
Hirschmann, Jane R.and Munter, Carol H., 1995, *When Women Stop Hating Their Bodies*, Reed Books Australia.
Orbach, Susie, 1998, *Fat is a Feminist Issue*, Arrow.

Other
Jo Anne Baker, author and proprietor of 'The Pleasure Spot' (specialises in workshops and private counselling in this field.

Festivals

NSW
Invoking the Goddess – Women's Spring Creation Gathering Four-day spiritual festival. Women only (very strong dyke presence), celebrating the great feminine Divine creative force – the Goddess within and without.

Workshops, rituals, entertainment and fabulous food in a glorious bushland setting. Tel: Anique Radiant Heart 02 9664 2714 or 0414 664270. Email: Anique@herwill.net. Webstite: www.herwill.net.

Sistajive – Women's Music Festival All information from Waves Music. Tel: 02 4268 3393.

Sydney Gay and Lesbian Mardi Gras Tel: 02 9557 4332. Website: http://www.mardigras.com.au/SGLMG.html.

Sydney Women's Festival Website: http://www.sydneywomensfestival.com.

Lesfest The organising committee changes from year to year. Get *LOTL* or *Lesbian Network* and keep an eye out for the ads. Fantastic wimmin's space.

QLD

Brisbane Pride Collective PO Box 5159, West End, Qld 4101. Tel: Cath: 0418 152 801. Email: cnspride@hotmail.com. Website: www.pridebrisbane.org.au.

VIC

Midsumma Festival Inc. 1st Floor, Fitzroy Town Hall, Napier St, Fitzroy, Vic 3065. PO Box 2248, Fitzroy Business Centre, Vic 3065 Tel: 03 9415 9819. Fax: 03 9415 9817. Email: admin@midsumma.org.au. Website: www.midsumma.org.au/.

SA

Feast – Adelaide Lesbian and Gay Cultural Festival PO Box 8183, Station Arcade, Adelaide, SA 5000. Tel: 08 8231 21 55. Fax: 08 8251 8793. Email: feast@feast.org.au. Website: www.feast.org.au/perpetual/contact.php.

WA

Pride Festival (Lesbian and Gay Pride WA Inc.) PO Box 30, North Perth, WA 6906. Tel: 08 9227 1767. Email: pride@pridewa.asn.au.

International

The Michigan Womyn's Music Festival. August every year. Website: http://www.michfest.com/home.html.

Health

Books

Blum, Jeanne Elizabeth, 1995, *Woman Heal Thyself: An Ancient Healing System for Contemporary Women*, Element Books.

Brownworth. Victoria A., 2000, *Coming out of Cancer: Writings from the Lesbian Cancer Epidemic*, Seal Press.

Hardin, Kimeron and Hall, Marny, 2001, *Queer Blues: The Lesbian and Gay Guide to Overcoming Depression*, New Harbinger Publications.

The Boston Women's Health Collective, 1984, *The New Our Bodies, Ourselves*, Penguin Books (dated, out of print, but still full of really good information).

The Boston Women's Health Book Collective, 1998, *Our Bodies, Ourselves: For the New Century*, Touchstone/Simon & Schuster.

The Federation of Feminist Women's Health Centres, 1981, *A New View of a Woman's Body*, Simon & Schuster, Inc. 1991–1996, Feminist Health Press.

Nissim, Rina, 1984, *Natural Healing in Gynaecology: A Manual for Women*, Pandora.

Northrup, Christiane, MD, 1998, *Women's Bodies, Women's Wisdom*, Bantam Books.

White, Jocely, C. and Martinez, Marissa C., 1997. *The Lesbian Health Book – Caring for Ourselves*, Seal Press.

Other

GLBT Health Access Project: This organisation has developed standards of practice for the provision of health care to GLBT clients and their families. They have also developed 'Homophobia in health care is unhealthy' posters. Website: www.glbthealth.org.

Finding a health practitioner

As this book goes to press, the AIDS Council of New South Wales ('ACON', see p. 239) is working with the Australian Lesbian Medical Association and the Lesbian Health Interagency Network to create lesbian health resources. They are hoping to establish a database of lesbian-friendly health care professionals. They are also developing a resource to help lesbians get the best out of their health care workers. Other ACON services for women include a Women and HIV Team, counselling services and access to all HIV client care and support services.

NSW Lesbian Health Interagency Network is a group of organisations and individuals committed to improving and promoting the health of lesbians and women who have sex with women. Contact through Jen Rudland at the AIDS Council of NSW (see p. 239).

Herpes

Books

Sacks, Stephen L., 1997, *The Truth About Herpes*, Gordon Soules Book Publishers Ltd.

Biro, George, 1995, *The Herpes Handbook*, Gore & Osment Publications, 150 Queens Street, Woollahra, NSW 2025.

Also see Northrup, C., under '*Health*', above.

Homophobia

Website http://www.stophomophobia.org

Immigration

Gay & Lesbian Immigration Task Force (NSW) 1st Floor, 94 Oxford Street (PO Box 400), Darlinghurst, NSW 2010. Tel: 02 9380 5950.
Fax: 02 9569 5959. Email: gltf@dot.net.au. Website: www.gltf.org.au.
Gay and Lesbian Immigration Task Force QLD (Inc.) PO Box 378,
Paddington, Qld 4064. Tel/Fax: Trevor 07 3367 0731;
Grant: 07 3855 3201. Email: info@glitf.powerup.com.au.
Website: http://www.glitf.powerup.com.au/.
GAY & LESBIAN IMMIGRATION TASK FORCE INC
Tel (secretary): 03 9853 6559, 03 9523 7864.
Email: glItfvic@hotmail.com. Website: www.glItf.gaybookings.com.

Intersex and androgynous people

An international email group for intersex and androgynous people can be contacted at Intersex-Androgynous@yahoogroups.com.

Lesbians and the law

Auckland Lesbian and Gay Lawyers Group PO Box 5918, Wellesley St, Auckland.
Acts of Passion Lesbians, Gay Men and the Law: a joint project of NSW Young Lawyers, Gay and Lesbian Rights Lobby, Inner City Legal Centre, NSW Attorney-General's Department and the AIDS Council of NSW. Available from AIDS Council of New South Wales (see p. 239).
Gay and Lesbian Rights Lobby Level 1, 94 Oxford Street (PO Box 9), Darlinghurst, NSW 2010. Tel: 02 9332 1966. Email: info@glrl.org.au. Website: http:rainbownet.au/~glrl/.
Gay and Lesbian Legal Rights Service This Sydney-based service operates from 6–10 pm on Wednesday nights only. Tel: 02 9332 1966.

Gala legal kits See the Gala website below. This national organisation provides free legal kits covering wills, power of attorney, and enduring guardianship and property agreements. Gala also provides a legal referral service.

Australian Lesbian Lawyers Tel: Caroline Marsh 02 9353 4646. Email: caro268@hotmail.com.

NSW

Women's Legal Resources Centre Tel: 02 9749 5533.

QLD

Women's Legal Service Tel: 07 3392 0670 or toll free 1800 816 349. TTY: 1800 670 864.

Sexuality and Gender Rights (Qld) Tel: 07 3357 1183, 0410 556 150. Website: www.Gaylawnet.com.

SA

Women's Legal Service Tel: 08 8221 5553 or 1800 670 864.

'You and the Law' Contact through the Gay and Lesbian Counselling Service.

TAS

Gay and Lesbian Rights Tel: 03 6224 3556.

VIC

Women's Legal Resource Group Tel: 03 9642 0943 or 1800 133302.

The Victorian Equal Opportunity Commission (see above) has a publication entitled 'Same Sex Relationships and the Law'. A preview of this document is available at http://www.eoc.vic.gov.au/publications/free/same_sex_relationships.htm.

WA

Women's Legal Service Tel: 08 9221 5122 or 1800 625 122.

Books

Monk, Daniel and Beresford, Sarah, 1998, *Legal Queeries: Lesbians, Gay and Transgender Legal Studies*, Cassell.

Women's Legal Resources Centre, 2000, *Lesbians and the Law: A Practical Guide*, 2nd ed., Redfern Legal Centre Publishing.

Lesbian lives

Books

Curb, Rosemary and Manahan, Nancy, 1985, *Lesbian Nuns Breaking Silence*, Bantam/Corgi Books.

Faderman, L., 1985, *Surpassing The Love of Men*, The Women's Press Limited.

Klaich, D., 1974, *Woman + Woman*, Simon and Schuster.

Mavor, E. 1971, *The Ladies of Langollen: A Study of Romantic Friendship*, Penguin Books.

Lesbian sex

Books

ACON, 1999, *The Informer: Lesbian Sex Revealed*, adapted from *Lesbian Sex* by Sarah Bergin, produced by Women's Campaigns.

ACON Women's Team, 1994, *Lesbian Sex*, AIDS and Infectious Diseases Branch of the NSW Department of Health.

Bright, Susie, 1990, *Susie Sexpert's Lesbian Sex World*, Cleis Press.

Caster, Wendy, 1993, *The Lesbian Sex Book*, Alyson Publications.

Dion, A. H., 1999, *The Strap On Book*, Greenery Press.

Johnson, S. E., 1996, *Lesbian Sex: An Oral History*, The Naid Press Inc.

Heart, Mikaya, 1994, *The Straight Woman's Guide to Lesbianism*, Tough Dove Books.

Loulan, J., 1984, *Lesbian Sex*, Spinsters Ink.

Lotney, Karlyn, 2000, *The Ultimate Guide to Strap-On Sex. A Complete Resource for Women and Men*, Cleis Press.

Morin, Jack, 1981, *Anal Pleasure and Health*, Yes Press.

Newman, Felice, 1999, *The Whole Lesbian Sex Book: A Passionate Guide for All of Us*, Cleis Press.

Sisley E. and Harris, B., 1977, *The Joy of Lesbian Sex*, Simon & Schuster.

West, Celeste, 1989, *A Lesbian Love Adviser*, Cleis Press.

Schram-Evans, Zoe, 1995, *Making Out*, Pandora.

Lesbian women with disabilities

Access Plus Spanning Idenities This is a group of lesbian, gay, bisexual or transgender people with disabilities. Website: www.apsi.org.au. Contact APSI through People With Disabilities NSW (Inc.) Tel: 02 9319 6622. TTY: 02 9318 2138. Fax: 02 9318 1372 or write to Access Plus Spanning Identities, PO Box 520, Newtown, NSW 2042. Email: admin@apsi.org.au.

Deaf Gay and Lesbian Association (Victoria) Email: gla@primus.com.au.

Women With Disabilities Australia. (WWDA) PO Box 605 Rosny Park, Tas 7018. Tel: 03 6244 8288, 03 6253 5104. Fax: 03 6244 8255. Email: wwda@ozemail.com.au. Website: http://www.wwda.org.au.

Books

Tremain, Shelley, 1996, *Pushing the Limits – Disabled Dykes Produce Culture*, Ontario Arts Council.

Making babies and parenting

AIDS Council of NSW, *Talking Turkey: A Legal Guide to Self-Insemination*, Inner City Legal Centre (Tel: 02 9332 1966).
Peis, Cheri, 1988, *Considering Parenthood*. Spinsters Ink.
Pepper, Rachel, 1999, *The Ultimate Guide to Pregnancy for Lesbians: Tips and Techniques from Conception to Birth*, Cleis Press.

There are a number of other books. Please phone or write to the Feminist Bookshop (see above). They will be happy to send you their Babies & Parenting book list.

Masturbation

Books
Betty Dodson, 1996, *Sex for One: The Joy of Self-Loving*, Three Rivers Press.

Internet
Jillinworld www.geocities.com/Wellesley/Atrium/9135/page1.htm
Joy of masturbation www.bettydodson.com/subjoy.htm
Solo www.proaxis.com/~solo/
The Clitoris www.geocities/~debbie_fox/
The ultimate masturbation site
www.geocities.com/Wellesley/Atrium/9135/page1.html

Media

Internet
Dreadedned. www.dreadedned.com.au/source/groups/wa/support.htm
Provides links to many of the groups that exist in WA.
GALA http://www.gala.net.au/ Australia's Gay and Lesbian Alliance web page.
Gay.com http://gay.com Large, professional, informative.
Gay
Gay Australia Guide gayaustraliaguide.bigstep.com
Girlfriends http://www.gfriends.com Just a bit of light relief.
NZ Sites New Zealand's 100 per cent lesbian guide: lesbian.co.nz
Queer Resources online guide qrd.org.nz
Out Biz http://www.outbiz.com. Gay and lesbian lifestyle and entertainment site.

Pink Sofa www.thepinksofa.com Personals: women seeking women, relationship/friendship. Lesbian-operated. Well run. Fun.
Pinkboard PINKBOARD. http://www.pinkboard.com.au/cgi/Personals Australian. Pink Board Personals: PLANETOUT http://planetout.com
Pink Pages www.pinkpages.net.nz
Pride Links www.pridelinks.com
Rainbow Happenings www.rainbowhappenings.com. An Australian 'What's On' and accommodation directory.
Rainbow.Net www.home.rainbow.net.au/ Australian gay and lesbian Internet service provider.
Rainbow Network http://www.rainbownetwork.com/
Qpages WA Gay and Lesbian Business Directory. http://www.qpages.com.au

Chat rooms
Gay.com www.gay.com
Lesbian chat galore www.4wmn.com
Pink Sofa www.thepinksofa.com

Print
NSW
Lesbians on the Loose. Full of information about what's on; ads for lesbian businesses and services; contact lists for lesbian community and social groups. Tel: 02 8347 1033. Fax: 02 9380 6529. Email: lotl@lotl.com. PO Box 1099, Darlinghurst, NSW 1300 (*LOTL* is mailed in a plain envelope to protect your privacy.) Website (with contact and dating service): http://www.lotl.com.
Mountain Lesbian News Blue Mountains magazine PO Box 2, Katoomba, NSW 2780. Tel: 02 4751 2578.
Sydney Star Observer Great gay community newspaper. More gay than lesbian. Can be purchased in many Sydney newsagencies. Tel: 9380 5577. Website: http:www.ssonet.com.au. Website: www.SSO.com.au.
What's On For Women (WOW) Northern Rivers region magazine. Tel: 02 6621 5080 (ah).Website: www.wow@lis.net.au.
QLD
Queensland Pride Newspaper All lesbian, gay, bisexual and transgender issues throughout Queensland. Subscribe or buy at selected outlets (gay venues and adult shops). PO 8151, Woolloongabba, Qld 4102. Tel: 07 3392 2922. Email: Qldpride@powerup.com.au. Contacts: Catherine McKenzie, Women's editor, Iain Clacher, newseditor.
QNews Tel: 07 3852 5933. Email: Ray@qnews.com.au.

SA

Blaze Gay community newsletter. PO Box 10255, Adelaide Business Centre, Adelaide, SA 5000. Tel: 08 8211 9199. Fax: 08 8211 7399. Email: editor@blazemedia.com.au. Website: www.blazemedia.com.au.

Liberation Women's Studies Resource Centre, 64 Pennington Tce, North Adelaide, SA 5006. Women's liberation newsletter that has lesbian content.

TAS

I would suggest that Tasmanian lesbians consider subscribing to *Lesbiana* (see below). This magazine has Tasmanian content and listings.

VIC

Lesbiana Monthly magazine. PO Box 127, Kingsville, Vic 3012. Tel: 03 9687 3896, 0402 288 465.Email: lesbiana@primus.com.au.

WA

Grapevine PO Box K788, Perth, WA 6001. Tel: 08 9444 2989. Email: grapevine@technodyke.com.

Women Out West Magazine Website: http:/www.womenoutwest.com.au, http://www.womenoutwest.com.au/lesbianperth/links.shtml.

National

Lesbian Network PO Box 1338, South St Kilda, Vic 3182. Tel/Fax: 03 9525 7578. Email: Lesbian_net@hotmail.com.

Waves Music Newsletter PO Box 336, Thirroul, NSW 2515. Email: migwaves@hotkey.net.au.

New Zealand

The Tamaki Makaurau Lesbian Newsletter PO Box 44056, Pt Chevalier, Tamaki Makarau/Auckland 1002. Tel: 64 9 376 2454. Email: tminnews@voyager.co.nz. Website: womenz.org.nz/tmln.

Note The following fantastic website will link you up with most of the women's resources in NZ: www.womenz.org.nz.

Further Afield

There are two international magazines held by some Australian specialty bookshops.

Bad Attitude PO Box 39110, Cambridge MA 02139. Lesbian fiction, S/M.

Off Our Backs. 2337B 18th St, Washington DC 20009. Email: offourbacks@compuserve.com. Website: www.igc.org/oob.

On Our Backs Lesbian erotica. HAF Enterprises, Ste. 101, 3415 Cesar Chavez, San Francisco CA 94110. Email: staff@gfriends.com. Website: gfriends.com/onourbacks. Lesbian erotica.

Radio and TV

Dykes on Mykes 4ZZZ 102.FM. Alternate Wednesdays 7 pm–9 pm.

Gay Radio in Cyberspace http://gaydarradio.com

Gaywaves (2SER) Tel: 02 9514 9500.
Gaywaves Newcastle Tel: 049 215 555.
Gaywaves Northern Rivers Tel: 066 293 929.
Joy 90.7 FM Melbourne. On air Saturday to Tuesday each week.
Lesbian Radio Christchurch Plains 96.9 FM Monday 9 pm.
Out FM 94.5. Website: http:www.outfm.com.au.
Bent TV, Melbourne. Monday 9 pm, UHF Channel 13.
Pride TV, Perth. Tuesday 9.30 pm, Saturday 11 pm, Channel 31.

Menopause

Books

Allen, R., 1994, *HRT – Is It for Me?*, The Health Book Series, Gore & Osment Publications, Private Box 427, 150 Queen Street, Woollahra, NSW 2025.

Andrews, Lynn V., 1993, *Woman at the Edge of Two Worlds: The Spiritual Journey Through Menopause*, Harper Perennial.

Andrews, Lynn V., 1994, *Woman at the Edge of Two Worlds: Workbook: Menopause and the Feminine Rites of Passage*, Harper Perennial.

Doress-Worters and Siegal, 1994, *The New Ourselves, Growing Older: Women Aging with Knowledge and Power*, Touchstone/Simon & Schuster.

Farrell, E., Dec 1999, 'Hormone Replacement Therapy – Current Prescribing Choices', *Australian Family Physician*.

Greer, Germaine, 1991, *The Change*, Hamish Hamilton Ltd.

Kenton, Leslie, 1998, *Passage to Power: Natural Menopause Revolution*, Random House.

Sundquist, K., 1992, *Menopause – Make it Easy, The Health Book Series*, Gore & Osment Publications, Private Box 427, 150 Queen Street, Woollahra, NSW 2025.

Weeds, Susan, 1992, *Menopausal Years: The Wise Woman's Way: Alternative Approaches from Women*, Ash Tree Publishing.

Slayton, Tamara, 2000, *Reclaiming the Menstrual Matrix: Evolving Feminine Wisdom*, Lantern Books.

Lynch, Lee and Woods, Akia, 1996, *Off the Rag: Lesbians Writing on Menopause*, New Victoria Press.

Nelson, Mariam E., 1997, *Strong Women Stay Young*, Thomas C Lothian Pty Ltd, Bantam.

Northrup, C., 1998, *Women's Bodies, Women's Wisdom*, Bantam Books.

Northrup, C. 2001, *The Wisdom of Menopause*, Piatkus.

Sang, Barbara, Warshow, J. and Smith, Adrienne J. (eds), 1991, *Lesbians at Midlife: The Creative Transition*, Spinsters Book Co.

Older lesbians

NSW

JJ's Ballroom Dancing. All ages. Greatly enjoyed by lots of older dykes.
Tel: 02 9363 4735.

10/40 Matrix Social and political group for feminists over 40. Organises
national conferences. PO Box 142, Camperdown, NSW 1450. Tel: 02 9810
5130. Website: www.olderdykes.org.

Mature Aged Dykes Middle Aged Gals (MADMAGS) Social group that
meets monthly for coffee. Tel: 02 9799 3450.

'Older Lesbians Out and About' regular column in *Lesbians on the Loose* (see
'Media' above).

Over 45 Social Group Tel: 02 9817 5304.

OWLS Older (35 and over), wiser lesbians. PO Box 610, Petersham, NSW
2049.

Contact people in these organisations are extremely welcoming. Don't let the
fact that you are by yourself hold you back. Make the phone call and take
the step. You often get to know more people when you are by yourself. Also,
consider Clover Club, Black & White Dinner Dances, Leaders and Followers
Dinner Dances (see *LOTL* for details).

QLD

OWLS Older, wiser lesbians. PO Box 10106, Adelaide St, Brisbane, Qld
4000. Email: brisowls@mail.com. Website: www.geocities.com/brisowls.

SA

Lesbian Matriarchs PO Box 38, Inman Valley, SA 5211.
Tel/Fax: 08 8558 8376. Email: cann@chariot.net.au.

VIC

Matrix Guild Victoria Inc. PO Box 99, Fairfield, Vic 3078.

If you do not find a group in your state listed here, I would strongly suggest
that you subscribe to *Lesbian Network* in order to access the contact list
published by this magazine.

Parents of lesbians

PFLAG (Parents and Friends of Lesbians and Gays)

ACT

Make contact through **Gay Information and Counselling Service ACT**,
GPO Box 229, Canberra, ACT 2061. Tel: 02 6247 2726. Fax: 02 6257 4838
or Margaret 02 6251 1599 or Pat: 02 6242 0590.

NSW

NSW Information Line Tel: (02) 9294 1002. In NSW, PFLAG groups exist in Albury, Bathurst, Campbelltown, the Central Coast, Gunnedah/Tamworth, the Illawarra, the Northern Rivers region, Port Macquarie, the Murray Irrigation Area (Griffith) and Wagga Wagga as well as Sydney and Western Sydney. Contact details can be obtained from the main NSW Information line, or from the PFLAG Western Sydney
Website:http://www.pflagwestsyd.org.au/

TAS

12 Derwent Waters, Claremont, TAS 7011. Tel: Carol/Doug 03 6249 5778.

VIC

Information and helpline: 03 9511 4083.
Website: www.geocities.com/westhollywood/6076/. As well as Melbourne, PFLAG has groups at Geelong and Sunrasia (phone Melbourne group for information).

QLD

Brisbane: Shelley 07 3017 1739, (m) 0409 363 335. Email:
pflagbus@hotmail.com. Website: pflagbrisbane.com.
Sunshine Coast: (07 5450 6332). Website: www.geocities.com/pflagscoast.

SA

PO Box 4018, Seaton, SA 5023. Tel: Pam 08 8241 0616, Ralph 08 8369 0718. Fax: 08 8369 0718. Email: pamandon@tpg.com.au. Also:
ralph@tpg.com.au. Web site: www.pspflag.asm.au.

WA

102 Aberdeen St, Northbridge, WA 6003. Tel: 08 9228 1005.
Fax: 08 9228 1006.Email: pflagperth@telstra.easymail.com.au.
Website: http://www.pflag.org.au.
Email support list: http://www.critpath.org/pflag-talk/.

2010 Youth Centre

2010 is a youth service dedicated to working with young lesbian women and gay men to prevent homelessness. They can help link you up with work, training and education. Any lesbian young woman is welcome to contact them. The families of gay and lesbian young people may also use this service. They provide support, information and links to networks.
Tel: 02 95526130 or 1800 65 2010. Email: twenty10@rainbow.net.au.
Website: http://www.rainbow.net.au/~twenty10/.

Websites

My Child is Gay http://www.pe.net/~bidstrup/parents.htm
Pflag USA http://www.pflag.org
The coming out of a lesbian mother
http:/www.angelfire.com/co/lesmom/index/htm (very useful)

Politics

Organisations
Coalition of Activist Lesbians (COAL) PO Box 424, Thirroul, NSW 2515.
Website: www.Coal.zip.com.au. COAL has produced three wonderful
resources: 'Out for Justice', 'Out for Our Lives', 'Out for Our Sisters'. They
have also produced position papers and 'An Overview of Lesbians and Health
Issues'.
GALE (Gay and Lesbian Equality WA) PO Box 420, Northbridge, WA
6865. Tel: 08 9272 4515. Email: galewa@galewa.asn.au.
Website: www.galewa.queer.org.au.

Books
Willet, G., 2000, *Living Out Loud: A History of Gay and Lesbian Activism in
Australia*, Allen & Unwin.

Websites
http://www.queertheory.com – QueerTheory.com provides online integrated
visual and textual resources in Queer Culture, Queer Theory, Queer Studies,
Gender Studies and related fields.

Reference and research

Organisations
The Lesbian Health Research Network Email: r.mcnari@unimelb.edu.au
Australian Centre for Lesbian and Gay Research. Building H31,
University of Sydney, NSW 2006. Tel: 02 9351 5561. Fax: 02 9351 5562.
Email: aclgr@social.usyd.edu.au.
Australian Research Centre for Sex Health and Society Latrobe University,
Locked Bag 12, Carlton South, Vic 3053.

Books
Alexander, Christopher J. (ed.), 1996, *Gay and Lesbian Mental Health: a Source
Book for Practitioners*, Harrington Park Press.
Cabaj R. P. and Steil T. S. (eds), 1999, *Textbook of Homosexuality and Mental
Health*, American Psychiatric Press, Inc.
Davies, Dominic and Neal, Charles, 1999, *Kink Therapy. A Guide for
Counsellors and Therapists. Working with Lesbian, Gay and Bisexual Clients*,
Open Uni Press.
Jagose, Annamarie, 1996, *Queer Theory*, Melbourne University Press.

Relationship issues

Books
Leonhard, Gwen and Mast, Jennie, 1997, *Feathering Your Nest: An Interactive Workbook and Guide to a Loving Lesbian Relationship*, Rising Tide Press.

Berzon, Betty, 1990, *Permanent Partners: Building Gay and Lesbian Relationships That Last*, Plume (Penguin Group).

Loulan, JoAnn, 1987, *Lesbian Passion – Loving Ourselves and Each Other*, Spinsters/AuntLute Book Company.

Renzetti, Clare M. and Miley, Charles Harvey, 1996, *Violence in Gay and Lesbian Domestic Partnerships*, Harrington Park Press.

McNab, Claire and Gedan, Sharon, 1997, *The Loving Lesbian*, The Naid Press.

Search engines and email lists for lesbian issues

Search engines
http://www.cybersocket.com
http://www.bglad.com
http://www.gaycrawler.com
http:www.pridelinks.com
http:www.gayzoo.com
http:www.gayscape.com

Lists
International G/L/B/T Groups
http://www.rainbow.net.au/~glrl/International_GLBT_Groups.htm

Self-esteem

Books
Atkinson, Sue, 2001, *Building Self-Esteem*, Lion Publishing.

Cooke, Kaz, 1997, *Real Gorgeous*, Allen and Unwin.

Field, Lynda L., 2001, *Self-Esteem for Women*, Vermilion Publications.

Field, Gael Linden, 2000, *Self-Esteem: Simple steps to develop self-worth and heal emotional wounds*, Thorsons.

Sex addiction

Books
Davis Kasl, Charlotte, 1989, *Women, Sex and Addiction*, HarperCollins.
Melody, Pia and Wells, Andrea, 1992, *Facing Love Addiction*, HarperCollins.
Wilson-Schaef, Anne, 1998, *Escape From Intimacy: Untangling the Love Addictions, Sex, Romance, Relationships*, HarperCollins.
See also the books listed under 'Addiction' on p.234.

Sexual assault

NSW
Dymphna House Child Sexual Assault Counselling & Resource Centre
(including support for adult surviviors of CSA), PO Box 22, Haberfield, NSW 2045. Tel: 02 9797 6733, 02 9716 5100, Freecall 1800 654 119.
QLD
Rape Crisis Centre (Brisbane) Tel: 07 3391 0004.

Many regional health services now offer sexual assault counselling. Ring the hospital switchboard and ask for the sexual assault counsellor.

Books
Bass, Ellen and Davis, Laura, 1981, *The Courage to Heal: A Guide for Women Survivors of Child Sexual Abuse*, Harper & Row.
Davis, Laura, 1990, *The Courage to Heal Workbook: For Women and Men Survivors of Child Sexual Abuse*, Harper & Row.
Davis, Laura, 1991, *Allies in Healing – When the Person You Love Was Sexually Abused as a Child*, HarperCollins.
Haines, Staci, 1999, *The Survivor's Guide to Sex – How to Have an Empowered Sex Life After Child Sexual Abuse*, Cleis Press.
Maltz, Wendy, 2001, *The Sexual Healing Journey – A Guide for Survivors of Sexual Abuse*, Quill.

Sex and spirituality

Books
Levine, S. and O., 1995, *Embracing the Beloved: Relationship as a Path to Awakening*. Doubleday. Heterosexual, and more about relationships than sex, but very useful nevertheless.

Mariechild, Diane and Martica, Marcelina, 1995, *Lesbian Sacred Spirituality*,
    Wingbow Press. A most beautiful book!

Websites
www.tantra.org/lesbian.html
www.tantra.org/

Spirituality generally

NSW

Acceptance Sydney Gay & Lesbian Catholics. PO Box K222, Haymarket,
NSW 1240. Tel: 02 9568 4433. Email: acceptsyd@yahoo.com. Website:
http://sites.netscape.net/acceptsyd.

Buddhist Buddhist Library and Education. Tel: 02 9519 6054.

Heart Centre Susan MacFarlane and Georgia Carr facilitate daily Living
Awareness Circles and Residential Retreats which include meditation, music,
sharing, and teachings on the integration of love into daily life. HeartCentre,
Inspiration Place, Berrilee, NSW 2159. Tel: 02 9655 1055.
Email: heartc@zeta.org.au. Website: heartcentre.com.au.

Invoking the Goddess Women's Spring Creation Gathering See 'Festivals'
for more information about the dyke spiritual event of the year.

Jewish Outreach Tel: Michael 02 9300 9700.

Metropolitan Community Church Rev Greg Smith. 96 Crystal Street,
Petersham, NSW 2049. Tel: 02 9569 5122. Website:
http://www.mccsydney.org.au.

Metropolitan Community Church of the Good Shepherd (Parramatta) Rev
Robert Clark. Parramatta. Tel: 02 9638 3298. These two churches are
churches of a Christian denomination with a positive and affirming outreach
to the gay, lesbian, bisexual and transgender communities. They are not
associated with any other Christian denomination. They state that they are
the world's largest gay and lesbian organisation, with churches in 18
countries. They have been established for 35 years.

The Open Door A church for gay and lesbian people in the greater west of
Sydney – 'where you are accepted for who god has created you to be'. Tel:
Sue 02 4730 4833, 04 3843 4735.

The Uniting Network (Uniting Church) PO Box 98, Enmore, NSW 2042.
Website: http:www.Adelaide.net.au/tildwmaster/un.

Quakers Religious society of Friends Tel: 02 9958 3322.

Queer Young Christians Tel: Jo 0410 597 536.

QLD

Metropolitan Community Church Tel: 07 3891 1388.
Email: pastor@mccbris.asn.au.
VIC
Acceptance Melbourne Inc. Gay & Lesbian Catholics. Tel: 03 9748 5688.

Books

Hodge, Dino, 1996, *The Fall Upward; Spirituality in the Lives of Lesbian Women and Gay Men*, Little Gem Publication.

Huerta, Christina, Jeremy P. Tarcher, 1999, *Coming Out Spirituality. The Next Step*, Putnam.

McCall Tigert, Leanne, 1996, *Coming Out While Staying In – Struggles and Celebrations of Lesbians, Gays and Bisexuals in the Church*, United Church Press.

Stuart, Elizabeth, 1996, *Just good friends. Towards a Lesbian and Gay Theology of Relationships*, Mowbray.

Transgender issues

ACT

Transgender Outreach PO Box 4707, Kingston, ACT 2604.
Tel: 0407 264 155.
NSW
The Gender Centre For specific information about transgender people and their concerns. Tel: 02 9569 2366, Website: www.gendercentre.org.au.
Wollongong Tel: Tran 02 4226 1163.
TAS
Tasmanian Transgender Support Group PO Box 2150, Hobart, Tas 7001.
VIC
Transgender Victoria PO Box 762, South Melbourne, Vic 3205.
Tel: 03 9517 6613. Email: tgvvic@ivillage.com. Website:
www.vicnet.net.au/~victrans.
Transgender Liberation and Care PO Box 245, Preston,Vic, 3072.
Tel: 03 9517 1237. Email: transhb@vicnet.net.au.
QLD
Australian Transgenderist Support Assoc of Queensland PO Box 212, New Farm, Qld 4005.
The Gender Clinic 484 Adelaide Street, Brisbane, Qld 4000 (PO Box 484, New Farm, Qld 4005). Tel: 07 3227 8679.
SA
South Australian Transsexuals Support Group PO Box 907, Kent Town, SA 5071, or make contact through the Gay and Lesbian Counselling Service.

NZ
Agender New Zealand PO Box 27–560, Wellington, New Zealand.
Tel: 64 025 575 094.
Information is also available from the International Foundation for
Androgynous Studies.
Website: www.ecel.uwa.edu.au/gse/staffweb/fhaynes/IFAS_Homepage.html.
United Kingdom Intersex Society. Website: www.ukia.co.uk.

Books and Publications
Feinberg, Leslie, 1996, *Transgender Warriors: Making of History from Joan of
Arc to Dennis Rodman*, Beacon Press.
Halberstam, Judith, 1998, *Female Masculinity*, Duke University Press.
Ramsey, Gerald, 1999, *Transmen and FTMs Identities, Bodies Genders and
Sexualities*, University of Illinois Press.
Nataf, Zachary I., 1996, *Lesbians Talk Transgender*, Scarlett Press.
Ramsey, Gerald, 1996, *Transexuals: Candid Answers to Private Questions*,
Crossing Press.
Cameron, Loren, 1996, *Body Alchemy – Transsexual Portraits*, Cleis Press.
Bornstein, Kate, 1994, *Gender Outlaws: On Men, Women, and the Rest of Us*,
Vintage Books.
Feinberg, Leslie, 1993, *Stone Butch Blues*, Fire Brand Books.
Whittle, Stephen, 1998, *The White Book, A Really Indispensable Manual for
Inhabiting a Transmans Being*, Press for Change.
Polare: a magazine for people with gender issues Tel: 02 9569 1176. Email:
polare_editor@yahoo.com.au.

Websites
In addition to those set out above, the following website is very useful.
The homepage of Julie Elizabeth Peters: http://home.pacific.net.au/~janie/.

Violence

Lesbian and Gay Anti-Violence Project 9 Commonwealth St, Surry Hills,
NSW 2010. PO Box 350, Darlinghurst, NSW 1300. Tel: 02 9206 2066 or
1800 063 060. Fax: 02 9206 2069. Email: avp@acon.org.au.
Website: www.avp.org.au.
Australian Federal Police Gay and Lesbian Liaison Officer Tel: 02 6256
7777.
NSW Police Gay and Lesbian Liaison Officers – the NSW Police Service
established the first GLLO position in order to create of trust between the
gay community and the Police Service. They do not exist in all localities. To

contact a GLLO, tel: 02 9281 0000. (This is the central police switchboard.
Ask for your local GLLO or speak to Sue Thompson.) Website:
http://www.eagles.bbs.net.au/%7Egllos/index.html.

QLD
Police Liaison Task Force Info & Emergency Help Tel: 0419 768732.
Gay and Lesbian Liaison Officer. Tel: 07 3364 6464.
Email: lgbt@police.qld.gov.au. Website: www.police.qld.gov.au/lgbt.htm.

SA
Lesbian Domestic Violence Action Group Inc. Southern Women's
Community Health Centre, PO Box 437, Noarlunga Centre, SA 5168.
Tel: 08 8384 9555.

TAS
Police Gay and Lesbian Liaison Officer Tel: 03 6230 2111.

VIC
Police Gay and Lesbian Liaison Officer Tel: 03 9247 6666.

WA
Police Gay and Lesbian Liaison Officer Tel: 08 9356 0555.

South Australia does not have a GLLO position. The Northern Territory is in
the process of establishing a GLLO position as this book goes to press.

Young lesbians

Kids Help Line Tel: 1800 55 1800. Website: http://www.kidshelp.com.au/.

NSW
2010 Youth Centre 2010 is a youth service dedicated to work with young
lesbian women and gay men to prevent homelessness. They can help link
you up with work, training and education. Any young lesbian is welcome
to contact them. The families of gay and lesbian young people may also use
this service. Tel: 02 95526130 or 1800 65 2010. Email:
twenty10@rainbow.net.au.
Website: http://www.rainbow.net.au/~twenty10/.
Space Support Group for young gay, lesbian, bi and transgender people
between the ages of 12 and 20 from 6 pm to 8 pm on Tuesday night. Inner
West Sydney. Tel: 02 9516 2233.
Young and Proud. For young women up to 25. Tel: 0403 744861.
Email: youngandproud@hotmail.com.

TAS
Gay Youth Network Gay Information Line Box 818, Sandy Bay, Tas 7005.
Tel: 03 6234 8179.
Hobart Women's Health Centre Lesbian health worker. Tel: 03 6231 3212.

Working It Out LGBT support service.
Tel: Hobart 03 6234 6122, Burnie 03 6434 6474.

VIC
Generation Q Social and support group for same-sex attracted young people
to age 18. 354 Main Road West, St Albans, Vic 3021. Tel: 03 9364 3200.
Email: gsyouth@infoxchange.net.au.
Melbourne Youth Support Service For 15–25-year-olds. Lesbian and gay
friendly. Referral and information. Tel: 03 9614 3688. Fax: 03 9614 3622.

QLD
Prospect House For homeless lesbian, gay, bisexual, transgender people
under 25 years. Medium to long-term accommodation. Not crisis support.
PO Box 8278, Woolloongabba, Qld 4102. Tel: 07 3398 4222, 07 3846 2362.
Sisters of Venus Young women exploring and celebrating their sexuality.
Tel: Megan 07 3847 9633. Email: sistersof venus@yahoo.com.

SA
Ring the Gay and Lesbian Counselling Service.
Second Storey Youth Health Service Tel: 08 8232 0233.

WA
The Freedom Centre An information and drop-in centre for gay, lesbian,
bisexual, transgender and queer youth. Provides information, support,
pool table, comfortable couches, Iinternet access. 95 Stirling Street,
Northbridge, WA 6003. Tel: 08 9228 0354. Open: Wed–Fri: 3–9 pm, Sat:
12 midday–9 pm Email: info@freedom.org.au. Website:
http://www.freedom.org.au.

NZ
Rainbow Youth Youthline House, 13 Maidstone St, Ponsonby (PO Box 5426,
Auckland). Tel. 64 9 376 4155. Email: info@rainbowyouth.org.nz.

Websites
Even though your parents can track where you've been on the Internet,
sites like ReachOut! are general sites for all youth – it contains heaps of
useful fact sheets and contact details. Internet cafes provide access to the
Internet.
Cool page for queer teens http://www.pe.net/~bidstrup/cool.html
Eligh: http://www.elight.org
Gay/lesbian/bi teens http://gaylesteen.about.com/teens/gaylestteens/
Outproud hhtp://www.outproud.org/ A great site with coming out stories,
resources, role models and links to other relevant sites.
Outlink http://outlink.trump.net.au/ Website of Outlink Network, a site
funded by the Australian Human Rights and Equal Opportunity
Commission's Lesbian, Gay and Bisexual Rural Youth Network.
Planetout http://www.planetout.com

Reachout http://www.reachout.asn.au/home.jsp. A great Australian website for young people, with links to lots of fact sheets on being lesbian or bisexual.
Same-sex attracted youth web page
http:www.latrobe.edu.au/www/centstd/survey/SSAYHOME.html
Stophomophobia http://www.stophomphobia.org/
Mogenic http://mogenic.com/

For more sites see 'Youth Resources' on the CyberSocket Search Engine.

Books for young people

Central Coast Community Health Service, *An Intergalactic Guide to Relationships* (booklet for same-sex-attracted young people). Available from Central Coast Health Service Tel: 02 4320 2578.

Herdt, Gilbert (ed.), 1989, *Gay and Lesbian Youth*, Harrington Park Press.

Heron, Ann, 1995, *Two Teenagers in 20, Writings by Gay and Lesbian Youth*, Alyson.

Gray, Mary, 1999, *In your face – Stories from the lives of Queer Youth*, Harrington Park Press.

Macleaod, Mark, 1996, *Ready or Not. Stories of Young Adult Sexuality*, Random House.

Rashid, Norrina and Hoy, Jane (eds), 2000, *Girl 2 Girl: The lives and loves of young lesbian and biseuxal women*, Diva Books.

Shale, Erin, 1999, *Inside Out,* Bookman Press. Stories of both young people and famous people.

Sonie, Amy, 2000, *Revolutionary Voices, A multicultural queer youth anthology*, Alyson.

References for youth workers

Central Coast Community Health Service, *Quick Guide – Information for workers on young people, sexuality and suicide prevention*. Available from Central Coast Health Service Tel: 02 4320 2578.

De Crescinzo, Teresa, 1994, *Helping Gay and Lesbian Youth,– New Policies, New Programs, New Practice*, Harrington Park.

Hillier, Lynne, Dempsey, Deborah, Harrison, Lyn, Beale, Lisa, Matthews, Lesley and Rosenthal, Doreen, 1998, 'Writing Themselves In – A National Report on the Sexuality, Health and Well-Being of Same-Sex Attracted Young People', National Centre in HIV Social Research, Australian Research Centre in Sex, Health and Society, Faculty of Health Sciences, La Trobe University, Locked Bag 12, Carlton South, Vic 3053.

Hillier, Lynne, Harrison, Lyn and Dempsey, Deborah, 1999, 'Whatever happened to Duty of Care? Same-Sex Attracted Young People's Stories of

Schooling and Violence Sexualities and Schools', *Melbourne Studies in Education*, Vol 40 No 2.

Hillier, Lynne, Harrison, Lyn and Dempsey, Deborah, 'Gendered (s) Explorations Among Same-Sex Attracted Young People in Australia', *Journal of Adolescence*.

Unks, Gerald, 1995, *The Gay Teen. Educational Practice and Theory for Lesbian Gay and Bisexual Adolescents*, Routledge.

References

ACON Women's Team, 1994, *Lesbian Sex*, AIDS and Infectious Diseases Branch of the NSW Department of Health, Sydney.

American Psychiatric Association, 1994, *Diagnostic and Statistical Manual of Mental Disorders* (DSM – IV), 4th edition, American Psychiatric Association, Washington.

Australian Bureau of Statistics, 1997, *Crime and Safety*, Australian Government Publishing Service, Canberra.

Australian Bureau of Statistics, 1998, *Disability, Ageing & Carers, Summary of Findings*, Australian Government Publishing Service, Canberra.

Australian Bureau of Statistics, 1999, *Deaths*, Australian Government Publishing Service, Canberra.

Bancroft, J., 1983, *Human Sexuality and Its Problems*, Churchill Livingston, Edinburgh, London, Melbourne.

Barton, D. and Joubert, L., 2000, 'Psychosocial aspects of sexual disorders', *Australian Family Physician*, 29 (6): 527–31.

Bell, A. P. and Weinberg, M. S., 1978, *Homosexualities: A Study of DiversityAmong Men and Women*, Simon & Schuster, New York.

Bland, L., 1993, 'Purity, Motherhood, Pleasure or Threat? Definitions of Female Sexuality 1900–1970s' in Cartledge, S. and Ryan, J., *Sex and Love*, The Women's Press, London.

Cass, V., 1999, 'Sexual Orientation Identity Formation: A Western Phenomenon' in Cabaj, R. P. and Stein, T. S., *Textbook of Homosexuality and Mental Health*, American Psychiatric Press, Inc, Washington, pp. 227–51.

Caster, W., 1993, *The Lesbian Sex Book*, Alyson Publications, Los Angeles.

Coalition of Activist Lesbians, 1998, *Part 1: Out For Our Lives; Part 2: Out For Justice; Part 3: Out For our Sisters*, Bradfield Nyland Group, Sydney.

Coney, S., 1991, *The Menopause Industry*, Penguin, Auckland.

Costigan, K., Dec 1996, '$95,000 for national lesbian lobby group', *Lesbians On The Loose*, PO BOX 1099, Darlinghurst, NSW 1300, p.14.

Costigan, K., Dec 1997, 'Far from Over', *Lesbians On The Loose*, p. 11.

Daly, M., 1973, *Gyn/Ecology: The Metaethics of Radical Feminism*, Beacon Press, Boston.

Duncan, K., James, C. and Rodger, F., Jan 2000, 'Tenth Anniversary Special', *Lesbians On The Loose*, p. 14.

Dunne, S. (ed.), 1997, *1998 Sydney Gay & Lesbian Mardi Gras Festival Guide*, Sydney Gay & Lesbian Mardi Gras Limited, 21–23 Erskineville Rd, Erskineville, NSW 2043.

Dodson, B., 1996, *Sex for One – The Joy of Self-Loving*, Three Rivers Press, New York.

Edwards, A. and Thin, R. N., 1990, 'Sexually transmitted diseases in lesbians', *Int J STD AIDS*, 1:178–81 [Medline].

Faderman, L., 1985, *Surpassing The Love of Men*, The Women's Press Limited, London.

Farrelly, B., Feb 1997, 'Green, Gay and call me Giz', *Lesbians On The Loose*, pp. 3, 9 and editorial.

Farrelly, B. and Rand, F., April 1998, 'Your God shall be my God…', *Lesbians On The Loose*, p. 24.

Fethers, K., Marks, C., Mindel, A. and Estcourt, C. S., 2000, 'Sexually transmitted infections and risk behaviours in women who have sex with women', *Sexually Transmitted Infections*, 76: 345–49.

Gidycz, C. A., Coble, C. N., Latham, L.,and Layman, M. J., 1993. 'Sexual assault experience in adulthood and prior victimisation experiences', *Psychology of Women Quarterly*, 17: 151–68.

Goldmeier, D., Keane, F. E., Carter, P., Hessman, A, Harris, J. R. and Renton, A., 1997, 'Prevalence of sexual dysfunction in heterosexual patients attending a central London genitourinary medicine clinic', *Int J STD AIDS*, 8 (5): 303–306.

Guyton, A. C., 1998 ,*Textbook of Medical Physiology*,W. B. Saunders Company, Philadelphia.

Herbert, S. E., 1996, 'Lesbian Sexuality' in Cabaj, R.P. and Stein, T. S., *Textbook of Homosexuality and Mental Health*, American Psychiatric Press Inc., Washington.

Hillier, L., Dempsey, D., Harrison, L., Beale, L., Matthews, L. and Rosenthal, D., 1998, *Writing Themselves In – A National Report on the Sexuality, Health and Well-Being of Same-Sex Attracted Young People*, National Centre in HIV Social Research, Australian Research Centre in Sex, Health and Society, Faculty of Health Sciences, La Trobe University, Locked Bag 12, Carlton South, Vic 3053.

Hite, S., 1976, *The Hite Report*, Macmillan, New York.

Jagose, A., 1996, *Queer Theory*, Melbourne University Press, Melbourne.

Kaplan, H. S., 1981, *The New Sex Therapies*, Bruner-Mazell, New York.

Kaplan, H. S., 1979, *Disorders of Sexual Desire*, Simon & Schuster, New York.

Kinsey, A. C., Pomeroy, W. B. and Martin, C.E, 1948, *Sexual Behavior in the Human Male*, W. B. Saunders Company, Philadelphia.

Kinsey, A. C., Pomeroy, W. B., Martin, C. E. and Gebhard, P. H., 1953, *Sexual Behaviour in the Human Female*, Pocket Books, New York.

Kehoe, M., 1988, 'Lesbians over 60 Speak for Themselves', *Journal of Homosexuality*, 16 (3–4): 1–111.

Kenton, Leslie, 1996, *Passage to Power: National Menopause Revolution*, Vermilion, London.

Klaich, D., 1974, *Woman + Woman: Attitudes toward Lesbianism*, Simon & Schuster, New York.

Kricker, A., 1995, 'HRT and breast cancer', *Breast NEWS: Newsletter of the NHMRC National Breast Cancer Centre*, Vol. 1, No. 1.

Kuriansky, J. B. and Sharpe, L., 1981, 'Clinical and research implications of the evaluation of women's group therapy for anorgasmia: a review', *Journal of Sex & Marital Therapy*, 7(4): 268–77.

Levine, S. B., 1992, *Sexual Life, A Clinician's Guide*, Plenum Press, New York.

Levine, R. J., May 1998, 'Sex and the human female reproductive tract – what really happens during and after coitus', *Int J Impot Res*, Suppl 1: S14–21.

Levine, S. and O., 1995, *Embracing the Beloved: Relationship as a Path to Awakening*, Doubleday, New York.

Llewellyn-Jones, D., 1981, *EveryMan*, Oxford University Press, London.

Lock, M., 1998, 'Menopause: lessons from anthropology' *Journal of Psychosomatic Medicine*, 60 (4): 410–19.

Loulan, J., 1984, *Lesbian Sex*, Spinsters Ink, San Francisco.

Mariechild, D. and Martin, M., 1995, *Lesbian Sacred Spirituality*, Wingbow Press, Oakland.

Masters, W. H. and Johnson, V. E., 1966, *Human Sexual Response*, Little, Brown and Company, Boston.

Masters, W. H. and Johnson, V. E., 1979, *Homosexuality in Perspective*, Little Brown and Company, Boston.

Mavor, E., 1973, *The Ladies of Langollen: A Study of Romantic Friendship*, Penguin Books, New York.

McNair, R., 2000, 'Lesbian Sexuality: Do GPs contribute to lesbian invisibility and ill health?', *Australian Family Physician*, Vol. 29, No. 6, 514–16.

Nataf, Z. I., 1996, *Lesbians Talk Transgender*, Scarlett Press, London.

Nichols, M., 1988, 'Low Sexual Desire in Lesbian Couples' in Leiblum, S. and Soresn, R. C. (eds), *Sexual Desire Disorders*, Guilford, New York, pp. 387–412.

Northrup, C., 1998, *Women's Bodies, Women's Wisdom*, Bantam Books, New York.

O'Connell, Helen E., Hutson, John M., Anderson, Colin R. and Plenter, Robert J., 1998, 'Anatomical Relationship Between Urethra and Clitoris', *The Journal of Urology*, Vol. 159, 1892–97.

Pireneas, E., Oct 1995, 'A Cool Reception', *Lesbians On The Loose*, pp. 24–25.

Pitt, H., 1997, 'Church split emerges over lesbian leader', *Sydney Morning Herald*, 14 July.

Pertot, S., 1985, *A Commonsense Guide to Sex*, Angus & Robertson, North Ryde.

Rees, M. A., O'Connell, H. E., Plenter, R. J. and Hutson, J. M., 2000, 'The Suspensory Ligament of the Clitoris: Connective Tissue Supports of the Erectile Tissues of the Female Urogenital Region', *Clinical Anatomy* 13: 397–403.

Reid, S., King, M. and Watson, J., 1997, 'Sexual dysfunction in primary medical care: prevalence, characteristics and detection by the general practitioner', *J Public Health Med*, 19 (4): 387–91

Rich, A., 1980, 'Compulsory Heterosexuality and Lesbian Existence', *Signs* 5, No. 4, pp. 631–60.

Schramm-Evans, Z., 1995, *Making Out – The Book of Lesbian Sex and Sexuality*, HarperCollins, San Francisco.

Sisley, E. and Harris, B., 1977, *The Joy of Lesbian Sex*, Simon & Schuster, New York.

Skinner, C. J., Stokes, J., Kirlew, Y. et al., 1996, 'A case-controlled study of the sexual health needs of lesbians', *Genitourinary Medicine*, 72: 277–80.

The Boston Women's Health Collective, 1984, *The New Our Bodies, Ourselves*, Penguin Books, Ringwood.

The Federation of Feminist Women's Health Centers, 1981, *A New View of a Woman's Body*, Simon & Schuster, New York.

The Women's Library, 1999, 'The Women's Library', *Lesbian Network*, Issue 28, p. 42.

Tuiten, A., Van Honk, J., Koppeschaar, H., Cernaards, C., Thijssen, J. and Verbaten, R., 2000, 'Time course of effects of testosterone administration on sexual arousal in women', *Archives of General Psychiatry*, 57 (2): 149–56.

Walker, B. G., 1983, *The Woman's Encyclopedia of Myths and Secrets*, Harper & Row, San Francisco.

Willet, G., 2000, *Living Out Loud: A History of Gay and Lesbian Activism in Australia*, Allen & Unwin, Sydney.

Endnotes

Introduction

1   'Straight' is a colloquial term for 'heterosexual'. See the Glossary, p. 231.

Chapter 1

1   E. Shorter, 1975, *The Making of the Modern Family*, Basic Books, New York (especially Chapter III). L. Faderman, 1995, *Surpassing The Love of Men*, The Women's Press Limited, London.

2   Faderman 1995.

3   A. P. Bell and M. S. Weinberg, 1978, *Homosexualities: A Study of Diversity Among Men and Women*, Simon & Schuster, New York.

4   Throughout this book I use the terms 'lesbians' and 'lesbian women' interchangeably. For a brief discussion of my reasons, see the Glossary.

5   While some lesbians and heterosexual women find the word 'dyke' unpleasant, large numbers of lesbian women are very comfortable with it. For more information, see the Glossary.

6   D. Klaich, 1974, *Woman + Woman: Attitudes toward Lesbianism*, Simon & Schuster, New York.

7   See the Glossary for a definition of 'Herstory'.

8   Klaich 1974.
9   Ibid.
10 Ibid.
11 Faderman 1995.
12 Ibid.
13 Ibid.
14 Ibid., p. 135.
15 E. Mavor, 1975, *The Ladies of Langollen: A study of Romantic Friendship*, Penguin, New York.
16 Faderman 1995, p. 124.
17 Ibid., p.122.
18 Ibid., pp. 137–38.
19 Ibid., pp. 74–84.
20 Ibid., p. 190.
21 Ibid., p. 370.
22 Ibid.
23 Faderman 1995, p. 241, referring to Krafft-Ebing, *Psychopathia Sexualis*, 1882.
24 G. Willet, 2000, *Living Out Loud: A History of Gay and Lesbian Activism in Australia*, Allen & Unwin, Sydney, p. 107.
25 Ibid., p. 105.
26 Ibid., p. 37.
27 K. Duncan, C. James and F. Rodger, Jan 2000, 'Tenth Anniversary Special', *Lesbians On The Loose*, p. 14.
28 S. Dunne (ed.), 1997, *1998 Sydney Gay & Lesbian Mardi Gras Festival Guide*, Sydney Gay & Lesbian Mardi Gras Limited, Erskineville.
28 Willet 2000.
29 S. B. Levine, 1992, *Sexual Life – A Clinician's Guide*, Plenum Press, New York.
30 ibid.
31 A. C. Kinsey, W. B. Pomeroy, C. E. Martin and P. H.Gebhard, 1953, *Sexual Behaviour in the Human Female*, Pocket Books, New York.
32 Ibid.
33 Ibid. D. Llewellyn-Jones, 1981, *EveryMan*, Oxford University Press, London.
34 The Boston Women's Health Book Collective, 1984, *The New Our Bodies, Ourselves*, Penguin Books, Ringwood.
35 S. Hite, 1976, *The Hite Report*, Macmillan, New York.
36 Ibid.
37 Faderman 1995.
38 The Boston Women's Health Collective 1984, p. 126.
39 C. A. Gidycz, C. N. Coble, L. Latham, M. Layman, M. A. Burnam et al., 1993, 'Sexual assault experience in adulthood and prior victimisation experiences', *Psychology of Women Quarterly*, 17: 151–1681, p.168.
40 Gidycz et al. 1993, p. 151.
41 Ibid., p. 152.
42 Ibid., p. 152.

Chapter 2
1   The Boston Women's Health Book Collective 1984.
2   The Federation of Feminist Women's Health Centers, 1981, *A New View of A Womans Body*, SImon & Schuster, New York.
3   Ibid., p. 33.
4   H. E. O'Connell, J. A. Hutson, C. R. Anderson and R. J. Plenter, 1998, 'Anatomical Relationship Between Urethra and Clitoris', *The Journal of Urology*, Vol. 159, p. 1892.
5   Ibid.
6   M. A. Rees, H. E. O'Connell, R. J. Plenter and J. M. Hutson, 2000, 'The Suspensory Ligament of the Clitoris: Connective Tissue Supports of the Erectile Tissues of the Female Urogenital Region', *Clinical Anatomy* 13: 397–403.
7   O'Connell 1998.
8   Rees et al. 2000.
9   The Federation of Feminist Women's Health Centres 1981, p. 39.
10 O'Connell et al. 1998.
11 See also p. 205 and Appendix 2, p. 214.
12 If you would like more details on how to do this, see The Boston Women's Health Collective 1984.
13 H. S. Kaplan, 1981, *The New Sex Therapies*, Bruner-Mazell, New York and H. S. Kaplan, 1979, *Disorders of Sexual Desire*, Simon & Schuster, New York.
14 J. Loulan, 1984, *Lesbian Sex*, Spinsters Ink, San Francisco, pp. 42–44.
15 Ibid., p. 43.
16 Ibid., p. 43.

Chapter 3
1   A. Rich, 1980, 'Compulsory Heterosexuality and Lesbian Existence', *Signs 5*, No 4, p. 648.
2   Ibid., pp. 650–51.

Chapter 4
1   S. E. Herbert, 1996, 'Lesbian Sexuality' in R. P. Cabaj and T. S. Stein, *Textbook of Homosexuality and Mental Health*, American Psychiatric Press Inc, Washington.
2   Ibid.
3   Ibid.
4   See Glossary, p. 232.
5   Z. Schramm-Evans, 1995, *Making Out – The Book of Lesbian Sex and Sexuality*, HarperCollins, San Francisco, p. 158.
6   J. Loulan 1984, p. 47.
7   ACON Women's Team, 1994, *Lesbian Sex*, AIDS and Infectious Diseases Branch of the NSW Department of Health, Sydney, p. 13.

Chapter 5
1 K. Fethers, C. Marks, A. Mindel and C. S. Estcourt, 2000, 'Sexually transmitted infections and risk behaviours in women who have sex with women', *Sexually Transmitted Infections*, 76: 345–49.
2 Ibid. The study sample was women who have sex with women (WSW). Sexual health researchers use this definition because this information is collected by some sexual health clinics. WSW may not define themselves as lesbian. They may define themselves as heterosexual, and have sex with women only occasionally, or be sex workers who have sex with women for money. They may be bisexual. Research into the transmission of STIs concentrates on sexual behaviour, rather than the way people define themselves.

Chapter 6
1 Herbert 1996, p. 728.
2 Herbert 1996, p. 729.
3 Herbert 1996, p. 728.
4 L. Bland, 1983, 'Purity, Motherhood, Pleasure or Threat? Definitions of Female Sexuality 1900 – 1970s' in S. Cartledge and J. Ryan, *Sex and Love*, The Women's Press, London, p. 23.
5 B. Dodson, 1996, *Sex for One – The Joy of Self-Loving*, Three Rivers Press, New York, pp. 3–7.
6 Kinsey 1953, p. 163.

Chapter 7
1 Kinsey 1953.
2 J. Bancroft, 1993, *Human Sexuality and Its Problems*, Churchill Livingston, Edinburgh, London, Melbourne.
3 R. J. Levine, May 1998, 'Sex and the human female reproductive tract – what really happens during and after coitus', *Int J Impot Res*, Suppl 1: S14–21.
4 A. C. Guyton, 1986, *Textbook of Medical Physiology*, W. B. Saunders Company, Philadelphia, p. 980.
5 Ibid.
6 The Federation of Feminist Women's Health Centres 1981.
7 O'Connell 1982.
8 Hite 1976.
9 Kinsey 1953.
10 S. Read , M. King, J. Watson, 1997, 'Sexual dysfunction in primary medical care: prevalence, characteristics and detection by the general practitioner', *J Public Health Med*, 19 (4): 387–91 and D. Goldmeier, F. E. Keane, P. Carter, A. Hessman, J. R. Harris and A. Renton, 1997, 'Prevalence of sexual dysfunction in heterosexual patients attending a central London genito-urinary medicine clinic', *Int J STD AIDS*, 8 (5): 303–306.
11 S. Pertot, 1985, *A Commonsense Guide to Sex*, Angus & Robertson, North Ryde, pp. 134–36.
12 Levine 1992, p. 39.

Chapter 8

1   Herbert 1996, p. 735.
2   Ibid.
3   American Psychiatric Association, 1994, *Diagnostic and Statistical Manual of Mental Disorders* (DSM – IV), 4th edition, American Psychiatric Association, Washington, pp. 496–99.
4   Pertot 1985, p. 70.
5   Ibid.
6   Loulan 1984, pp. 142–50.
7   M. Nichols, 1988, 'Low Sexual Desire in Lesbian Couples' in S. Leiblum and R. C. Soresn (eds), *Sexual Desire Disorders*, Guilford, New York, pp 387–412.
8   C. Northrup, 1998, *Women's Bodies, Women's Wisdom*, Bantam Books, New York, p. 555.
9   W. H. Masters and V. E. Johnson, 1966, *Human Sexual Response*, Little, Brown and Company, Boston, pp. 117, 238.
10 C. Northrup 1998.
    A. Tuiten, J. Van Honk, H. Koppeschaar, C. Cernaards, J. Thijssen and R. Verbaten, 2000, 'Time course of effects of testosterone administration on sexual arousal in women', *Archives of General Psychiatry*, 57 (2): 149–56.
11 Loulan 1984.
12 'Monogamy was considered important by at least three-quarters of lesbian women in most studies', Herbert 1996, p. 734.
13 Loulan 1984, p. 42.
14 S. and O. Levine, 1995, *Embracing the Beloved: Relationship as a Path to Awakening*, Doubleday, New York.
15 Ibid.
16 Pertot 1985, p. 90.
17 E. Sisley and B. Harris, 1977, *The Joy of Lesbian Sex*, Simon & Schuster, New York.
18 Herbert 1996, p. 732.
19 Loulan. 1984, p. 82.
20 Herbert 1996,. p. 733.
21 American Psychiatric Association 1994, p. 505.
22 J. B. Kuriansky and L. Sharpe, 1981, 'Clinical and research implications of the evaluation of women's group therapy for anorgasmia: a review', *Journal of Sex &Marital Therapy*, 7 (4): 268–77.
23 D. Barton and L. Jourbert, 2000, 'Psychosocial aspects of sexual disorders', *Australian Family Physician*, 29 (6): 527–31.

Chapter 9

1   Levine 1992, p. 24.
2   Levine 1992, p. 26.
3   Kinsey 1948, 1953.
4   Levine 1992, p. 28.
5   Levine 1992, p. 28.

6   V. Cass, 1999, 'Sexual Orientation Identity Formation: A Western Phenomenon' in R. P. Cabaj and T. S. Stein, *Textbook of Homosexuality and Mental Health*, American Psychiatric Press, Inc, Washington, pp. 227–51.
7   Cass 1999, p. 236.
8   Ibid., p. 240.
9   Ibid., p. 244.
10 Ibid., p. 245.
11 Ibid., p. 246.
12 Ibid., p. 246.
13 Ibid., p. 247.

Chapter 10
1   *Lesbians On The Loose* is a Sydney monthly magazine. It offers subscriptions Australia-wide, and also has a Queensland section. See the Resources section.
2   W. Caster, 1993, *The Lesbian Sex Book*, Alyson Publications, Los Angeles, p. 45.
3   LGBT: Lesbian, Gay, Bisexual, Transgender (see the Glossary).
4   PFLAG: Parents and Friends of Lesbians and Gays. See the Resources section for contact details.

Chapter 11
1   Barbara G. Walker, 1983, *The Womans Encyclopedia of Myths & Secrets*, Harper & Row, San Francisco, p. 523.

Chapter 12
1   Some women call themselves lesbian, some women call themselves gay, some women call themselves dykes. These words are defined in the Glossary. They are all used to refer to women who relate (emotionally or sexually) primarily to other women. Bisexual women relate to both women and men.
2   See footnote 1 above.
3   L. Hillier, D. Dempsey, L. Harrison, L. Beale, L. Matthews and D. Rosenthal, 1998, *Writing Themselves In – A National Report on the Sexuality, Health and Well-Being of Same-Sex Attracted Young People*, National Centre in HIV Social Research, Carlton South, p. 3.
4   Ibid.
5   Ibid., p. 49.
6   Ecstasy.
7   Marijuana, Cannabis.
8   'Eccy Tuesday': if you take ecstasy on the weekend, it is common to experience a profound psychological and physical low on Monday or Tuesday. Well known to those who use this substance. The long-term impact is not known.
9   Op. cit., p. 35. Hilier 1998.
10 Ibid.

Chapter 13

1 Australian Bureau of Statistics, 1998, *Disability Ageing and Carers, Summary and Findings*, Australian Government Publishing Service, Canberra.
2 Ibid.
3 Ibid.
4 Ibid.
5 Australian Bureau of Statistics, 1997, *Crime and Safety*, Australian Government Publishing Service, Canberra.
6 Northrup 1998.
7 Ibid., p. 517.
8 Ibid.
9 Ibid.
10 M. Kehoe, 1988, 'Lesbians over 60 Speak for Themselves', *Journal of Homosexuality*, 16 (3–4): 1–111.
11 American Psychiatric Association 1994, p. 505.
12 Kehoe 1988.
13 Northrup 1998.
14 Ibid., p. 516.
15 Ibid.
16 Ibid., p. 522.
17 S. Coney, 1991, *The Menopause Industry*, Penguin, Auckland.
18 Northrup 1998, pp. 545–46.
19 M. Lock, 1998, 'Menopause: lessons from anthropology', *Journal of Psychosomatic Medicine*, 60 (4): 410–19. Northrup 1998, pp. 545–46. A. Kricker, 1995, 'HRT and breast cancer', *Breast NEWS: Newsletter of the NHMRC National Breast Cancer Centre*, Vol. 1, No. 1.
20 Wilson, J, *A Change of Heart*, Australian Doctor 16 November 2001, p. 29.
21 Leslie Kenton, 1996, *Passage to Power: Natural Menopause Revolution*, Vermilion, London.
22 Ibid.
23 It has been suggested that this is because the large drug companies which market synthetic hormones have been able to fund research. As bioidentical hormones are not able to be patented, there are no large corporations with a financial interest in proving their efficacy. Hence, to date, adequate studies are not available.

Chapter 14

1 Coalition of Activist Lesbians, 1998, 'Out and Active Lesbians: Fact Sheet', *Out for Our Sisters*, Bradfield Nyland Group, Sydney, p. 26.
2 Ibid.
3 Eleni Pireneas, Oct 1995, 'A Cool Reception', *Lesbians On The Loose*, pp. 14, 24–25.
4 Ibid.

Chapter 15

1   Willet 2000, p. 37.
2   Ibid., p. 36.
3   Ibid., p. 33.
4   Ibid., p. 33.
5   Ibid., p. 17.
6   Ibid., p. 17.
7   Ibid., p. 17.
8   Duncan et al. 2000, p. 11.
9   Ibid.
10 Ibid., p. 13.
11 The Women's Library, 1999, 'The Women's Library', *Lesbian Network*, Issue 28, p. 42.
12 J. Bliss, 1999, 'Leaping off the Edge', *Lesbian Network*, Issue 28, p. 38.
13 Ibid., p. 54.
14 Willet 2000, p. 198.
15 Duncan et al. 2000, p. 17.
16 *Time*, 14 April 1997, front cover and pp. 66–72.
17 The Federation of Feminist Women's Heath Centers 1981.
18 K. Costigan, Dec 1996, '$95,000 for national lesbian lobby group', *Lesbians On The Loose*, p. 4.
19 Duncan et al. 2000, p. 17.
20 Ibid.
21 B. Farrelly, Feb 1997, 'Green, Gay and call me Giz', *Lesbians On The Loose*, p. 9, editorial and p. 3.
22 B. Farrelly, Aug 1997, 'Lesbian priest: "I am who I am"', *Lesbians on the Loose*, p. 4. H. Pitt, 1997, 'Church split emerges over lesbian leader', *Sydney Morning Herald*, 14 July.
23 Duncan et al. 2000, p. 19.
24 B. Farrelly, Dec 1997, 'Dorothy's friends...', *Lesbians On The Loose*, p. 7.
25 Ibid., p. 8.
26 Duncan et al. 2000, p. 19. K. Costigan, Aug 1997, 'Throwing open the closet door', *Lesbians On The Loose*, p. 6.
27 B. Farrelly and F. Rand, April 1998, 'Your God shall be my God...', *Lesbians On The Loose*, p. 24.
28 Ibid.
29 K. Costigan, Dec 1997, 'Far from Over', *Lesbians On The Loose*, p. 11.
30 Ibid., p. 13.

Appendix 2

1   The Federation of Feminist Women's Health Centers 1981, p. 39.
2   O'Connell 1998, p. 1896.

Appendix 3

1 K. Fethers, C. Marks, A. Mindel and C. S. Estcourt, 2000, 'Sexually transmitted infections and risk behaviours in women who have sex with women', *Sexually Transmitted Infections*, 76: 345–49.
2 Ibid.
3 Ibid.
4 'Head job'; oral stimulation of the penis sex. Also called ' fellatio'.
5 Op.cit. Feathers et al., 2000.
6 C. J. Skinner J. Stokes, Y, Kirlew et.al., 1996, 'A case-controlled study of the sexual health needs of lesbians', *Genito-urinary Medicine*, 72: 277–80.
   A. Edwards and R. N. Thin, 1990, 'Sexually transmitted diseases in lesbians', *Int J STD AIDS*, 1 :178–81 [Medline].

Glossary

1 *The Concise Oxford Dictionary*, Oxford University Press, 2000, Oxford.
2 Annamarie Jagose, 1996, *Queer Theory*, Melbourne University Press, Melbourne, p. 74.
3 M. Daly, 1973, *Gyn/Ecology: The Metaethics of Radical Feminism*, Beacon Press, Boston.
4 Jagose 1996, p. 72.
5 Ibid.
6 Ibid., p. 76.
7 Z. I. Nataf, 1996. *Lesbians Talk Transgender*, Scarlett Press, London.
8 Johnson 1996, p. 194.

Index